Dr Russ Harris is a medical practitioner, psychotherapist and psychologist who works in private practice, online teaching and the face to face training of counsellors and psychologists. He is also the best-selling author of *The Happiness Trap*, which has now been translated into 22 languages. Russ is one of the world's leading authorities on ACT, and regularly travels all over Australia as well as internationally to train a wide variety of professionals in the approach. His other books include *The Confidence Gap*, *ACT With Love*, *ACT Made Simple* and the fictional novel *Stand Up Strummer*. He lives in Melbourne.

Praise for *The Reality Slap*:

'As one of the world's pioneers of Acceptance and Commitment Therapy, Russ Harris has given us a truly compassionate gift on how to (en)lighten our journey through life's storms and calms. I had so many insightful moments that reading this book was a delight, an uplifting shoulder, and an education.'

— Professor Paul Gilbert, PhD, author of *The Compassionate Mind*

'Sooner or later, reality is going to slap you. Loss, disease, betrayal or other misfortunes will arrive unexpectedly and shake your very foundations. At that moment, this wise book is one to keep within reach. It will do more than soothe — it will ground you, guide you and help you grow. Taking the time to treat yourself with kindness and awareness doesn't remove the pain, but it dignifies it and turns it into a profound teacher. This book will help you learn the lessons that pain contains. You will want this book not just for you but also for those you love — knowing that sooner or later, reality is going to slap them too.'

— Steven C. Hayes, Foundation Professor of Psychology, University of Nevada, and author of *Get Out of Your Mind and Into Your Life*

'Deeply personal, profoundly insightful and above all highly practical, this book will show you how to deal with "Reality Slaps" — those painful wake-up calls that we all have when life is not fair or things go wrong. Russ Harris has produced another excellent book about what it means to be truly human, how to deal with life's difficulties, and how to live a more engaged, meaningful and pleasurable life.'

— Dr Anthony Grant, director, Coaching Psychology Unit, University of Sydney, and author of *8 Steps to Happiness*

'No matter what we attempt to do, pain and suffering are inevitably going to creep into our lives, and the capacity to handle this pain is essential for fulfilment. So if you want a short-term boost of happiness with simple, banal ideas that your kindergarten teacher could have told you, go elsewhere. But if you want to create a stable platform of mindfulness, meaning and purpose in your life, and develop the ability to handle pain effectively, then this is the book to read. It is my great hope that people will find this book and flexibly adopt the ideas within.'

— Dr Todd B. Kashdan, author of *Curious?* and *Designing Positive Psychology*

'Russ Harris is a world-renowned and highly respected trainer of Acceptance and Commitment Therapy, a modern scientific model of human psychology that overlaps to a great extent with aspects of traditional spiritual wisdom. In *The Reality Slap*, drawing from both scientific findings and his own personal experience, Russ invites us all into a vital conversation on how to handle life's tough edges. Read it, enjoy it, and you will find some genuine treasures in your life!'

— Dr Niklas Törneke, author of *The ABCs of Human Behaviour*

'Gripping, compassionate — a must-read for anybody going through a difficult life transition, such as divorce, illness, career change, or death of a loved one. This is a rare work, one that is at once deeply personal and universally applicable.'

— Dr Joseph Ciarrochi, Associate Professor, University of Wollongong, and author of *Emotional Intelligence in Everyday Life*

Also by Russ Harris

ACT Made Simple
ACT Questions and Answers
Act With Love
The Confidence Gap
Getting Unstuck in ACT
The Happiness Trap
The Weight Escape

THE REALITY SLAP 2ND EDITION:

How to survive and thrive when life hits hard

Russ Harris

ROBINSON

ROBINSON

First published in Australia in 2011 by Exisle Publishing Limited

First published in Great Britain in 2012 by Robinson

This edition published in 2021 by Robinson

3 5 7 9 10 8 6 4

Copyright © Russ Harris 2011, 2020

The moral right of the author has been asserted.

Note
This book is not intended as a substitute for medical advice or treatment.
Any person with a condition requiring medical attention should consult a
qualified medical practitioner or suitable therapist.

A CIP catalogue record for this book
is available from the British Library.

ISBN: 978-1-47214-636-6

Typeset in Adobe Jenson Pro by SX Composing DTP, Rayleigh, Essex
Printed and bound in Great Britain by Clays Ltd, Elcograf S.p.A.

Papers used by Robinson are from well-managed forests
and other responsible sources.

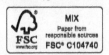

Robinson
An imprint of
Little, Brown Book Group
Carmelite House
50 Victoria Embankment
London EC4Y 0DZ

An Hachette UK Company
www.hachette.co.uk

www.littlebrown.co.uk

To my only child. When I wrote the first edition you were only five years old; and now, as I write the second, you are a young man of fourteen. In all the years I've known you, you have been by far my greatest teacher. Thank you for teaching me so much about living and loving; for helping me to grow and develop; for bringing so much joy and love into my life. I love you more than words can ever express

Contents

Part 1: Regroup

1: When life hurts   3

2: First things first   13

3: Kind words   23

4: Drop the struggle   37

5: When storms arise   45

6: Psychological smog   59

7: Notice and name   75

8: Live and let be   85

9: Our allies within   91

10: A curious look   101

11: A kind hand   115

12: When memories hurt   129

Part 2: Rebuild

13: Making life meaningful   143

14: One small step   161

15: The challenge formula   171

16: The prison of resentment   179

17: It's never too late   185

18: Breaking bad habits   191

Part 3: Revitalise

19: The stage show of life   205

20: The full experience   215

21: Joy and sorrow   223

Appendix A: Neutralisation   231

Appendix B: Mindfulness of the breath   237

Appendix C: Goal setting   241

Resources   247

Acknowledgments   251

Index   253

PART 1
REGROUP

1

WHEN LIFE HURTS

Nothing prepares you for those moments when reality slaps you in the face, sends you sprawling and turns your life upside down. A 'reality slap' can take many forms: the death of a loved one, a serious illness or injury, an horrific accident, divorce, betrayal, assault, infidelity, violent crime, job loss, bankruptcy, warfare, fire, flood, earthquake, pandemic ... and the list goes on. We don't like reality slaps, and we sure as hell don't want them — but sooner or later, if we live long enough, we're all going to have them. And one thing's for sure: the bigger the slap, the greater our pain. Depending on what we are facing, we may experience shock, sadness, anger, fear, anxiety, dread, guilt, shame — perhaps even hatred, despair or disgust. Indeed, sometimes the pain is so intense, so unbearable, our nervous system takes over and 'switches off our feelings', leaving us numb, empty or 'dead inside'.

Sometimes, if we're lucky, and the slap is not too forceful, we can recover fairly quickly. We can pick ourselves up, dust ourselves down, find a solution to the problem and carry on with our lives.

But what happens when there is no simple solution; when someone we love dies, or our partner leaves us, or we lose our job? If we sustain a major injury, develop a serious illness, experience a violent crime that wrecks our life? If our loved ones are sick or suffering? If the world falls into pandemic-induced chaos?

Reality slaps always involve loss. We may lose an important relationship — through death, divorce, separation or conflict. We may lose our health, or our job, or our independence. We may lose a sense of security, trust or safety. We may lose freedom, support, belonging — or many other things we deeply care about.

Reality slaps usually give rise to a crisis: a time of intense difficulty and uncertainty, where we're dealing with something awful over which we have little control. (This is especially likely with those life-crushing, soul-destroying reality slaps that psychologists refer to as 'trauma'.) At the same time, or very soon thereafter, comes grief. Contrary to popular belief, grief is *not* sadness; it is not an emotion at all. Grief is a psychological process of reacting to any significant loss. During a grieving process, we may feel a wide range of emotions from sadness and anxiety to anger and guilt, as well as physical reactions such as sleep disturbance, fatigue, lethargy, apathy and changes in appetite.

The five stages of grief

Dr Elisabeth Kübler-Ross famously described the 'five stages of grief' as denial, anger, bargaining, depression and acceptance. Although she was referring to death and dying, these stages apply to all types of loss, crisis and trauma. However, they are not discrete and well-defined stages — most people don't experience all of them, and there's no fixed order in which they occur. They tend to ebb and flow and blend into one another, and often they seem to 'end' but then 'start again'.

Whatever the nature of your loss, you are sure to experience at least some of these stages, so it's worth briefly discussing them.

'Denial' refers to a conscious or unconscious refusal or inability to acknowledge the reality of the situation. This could manifest as unwillingness to talk about it or think about it; or trying to pretend it's not happening; or a sense of being numb or 'shut down'; or a pervasive sense of unreality — walking around in a daze, feeling like it's all a bad dream. In the 'anger' stage, you might get angry with yourself, or others, or life itself. And anger's many close relatives frequently visit: resentment, indignation, fury, outrage, or a strong sense of unfairness or injustice.

'Bargaining' means attempting to strike deals that alter reality; this might include anything from asking God for a reprieve to asking a surgeon to guarantee the operation will be successful. It frequently involves lots of wishful thinking and fantasising about alternative realities: 'If only this had happened', 'If only that hadn't happened'.

The 'depression' stage is misnamed; it does not refer to the common clinical disorder known as depression. It refers to the emotions of sadness, sorrow, regret, fear, anxiety and uncertainty, which are natural human reactions to major loss.

Finally, the 'acceptance' stage refers to making peace with our new reality instead of struggling with it or avoiding it. This frees us up to invest our energy in gradually rebuilding our life (which right now may well sound impossible).

Fight, flight, freeze

Amidst all the chaos of a reality slap, we're going to experience some unpleasant physical reactions. We'll all experience the well-known 'fight-or-flight' response. And some of us will also experience the lesser known 'freeze' response.

To get a sense of what these responses are, why they happen and how they affect us, let's go on a journey backwards in time. Imagine one of our ancient ancestors is out by himself hunting rabbits, when suddenly he comes face to face with a huge mother bear. For a split second he freezes. The mother bear is fiercely protective of the two young cubs by her side; she sees the human as a threat — and she charges.

To survive this encounter, our ancestor has only two options: take flight or stay and fight. So, faster than the speed of conscious thought, his autonomic nervous system takes the helm. Now as you know, 'autonomy' means making your own decisions. And that's how the 'autonomic nervous system' gets its name — because it makes its own decisions about what's good for you, without any input from your conscious mind. So your mind doesn't go, 'Uh oh, better switch into fight-or-flight mode'. Your autonomic nervous system makes that decision for you before you even have time to register a thought; and it instantly revs up your body for 'fight or flight'.

So back to your ancient ancestor. Fight-or-flight mode kicks in. Large muscles in his arms and legs, chest and neck, tense up ready for action. His body floods with adrenaline and his heart speeds up, pumping blood to his muscles. He launches into fight mode, throwing his spear as hard as he possibly can.

But it's not a good throw. The spear only lightly grazes the bear and barely draws blood. The bear is now furious, and our ancestor has no other weapons. So he runs away as fast as he possibly can. Nothing matters now except escape.

But the mother bear is faster than the man. She catches him, knocks him to the ground.

There's no way the man can now fight off the bear and there's no possibility of running away. So again, faster than the speed of conscious thought, his autonomic nervous system takes control. Recognising that 'fight or flight' is no longer useful, the nervous system switches the body over to 'freeze'. Why? Because bears don't like their prey fighting back. So the more the man screams and struggles, the more viciously the bear will attack him. His best chance of survival is to lie as still and be as quiet as possible.

So this is where the 'freeze' response comes in. The vagus nerve (the second-largest nerve in the body, after the spinal cord) actively immobilises the man: it paralyses his muscles so he literally can't move. And at the same time it 'shuts off' the man's feelings. Why? Because the less pain he feels, the less he'll scream and struggle. So he lies there, literally 'frozen stiff', 'paralysed by fright', 'numb with fear'. If the man is lucky, then once he falls silent and lies still the bear might lose interest and go away, or he might survive long enough for someone to come and rescue him.

Our nervous systems and bodies are hard-wired to react in these ways — fight, flight or freeze — in response to any type of threat. (It's something we have in common with the nervous systems of all other mammals, as well as birds, reptiles and most types of fish.) Reality slaps are threatening, so when they occur we'll all have a fight-or-flight response. Most commonly this manifests as fear and anxiety (flight), but sometimes anger will predominate (fight). And in the most severe cases, if our nervous system perceives that fight or flight is futile, we'll go into freeze mode. If this happens to you, you may experience literally 'freezing up'; you can't move, can't speak. You may even 'black out' or have an 'out of body' experience.

In the days and weeks following a reality slap, fight, flight or freeze responses are likely to arise again and again. They are readily triggered by anything that reminds us of what we have been through;

this includes both things inside us — such as memories, thoughts, feelings and sensations — and things outside us, such as certain people, places, food, music, photographs, objects, books, news reports and so on. 'Fight' shows up as anger, frustration and irritability. 'Flight' shows up as fear, anxiety and worry. And 'freeze' shows up as numbness, apathy, tiredness, 'zoning out' or disengaging — and often feeds into a sense of futility, hopelessness, despair.

And now that we've touched on common reactions to reality slaps, the big question is …

What can we do about it?

The truth is, most of us don't cope well with reality slaps. We easily get 'hooked' by all those painful thoughts, feelings, memories and physical reactions; they jerk us around and pull us into self-defeating behaviours. For example, we might overuse drugs and alcohol, or withdraw from our friends and family, or drop out of activities we used to enjoy, or fight with the people we love, or hide away from the world, or spend way too much time in bed and on the couch.

All of these behaviours are normal — and extremely common. The problem is, they usually make things worse rather than better. But the good news is, we can change this state of affairs; we can learn new and more effective ways of responding to grief, loss and crisis. This book is based on an approach called Acceptance and Commitment Therapy, or ACT (which is said as the word 'act', not as the initials). ACT is a science-based approach, created by US psychologist Steven C. Hayes back in the 1980s. At the time of writing (2020), there are over 3000 studies on ACT published in top scientific journals, that demonstrate its effectiveness with everything from grief, depression and anxiety to addiction, chronic illness and trauma. It's a powerful and practical approach that helps people transcend their pain and suffering and build rich, meaningful lives despite adversity. And in the chapters that follow, I'll take you through it gently, step by step.

However, before we go any further, there are two points I really need to emphasise. First: there is no single 'right' or 'appropriate' reaction to a reality slap. Everyone reacts differently — so please let go of any preconceived ideas about what you should or shouldn't feel, and how long it should or shouldn't last. For example, some people cry for days and weeks on end, while others never shed a single tear; and both reactions are normal. Second: there is no single 'best' or 'correct' way to cope with grief, loss and crisis. Everyone copes differently, and what works for one person may not work for another. This book gives you lots of tips, tools, strategies and suggestions that have proven to be helpful for many people — but nothing works for everyone. So please: experiment, modify and adapt everything in this book to make it work for your unique situation and the challenges that go with it. (And that means dropping anything that *doesn't* work!)

By the time they get to my age (53) most people have experienced a fair number of reality slaps. Mine first started in childhood, with repeated abuse over many years from two close relatives. In later life, my reality slaps included the deaths of both parents, deaths of friends and family, a painful divorce, a major injury resulting in chronic pain, and an intensely stressful period of four years when my young son needed intensive ongoing treatment for a very serious condition. (To my great relief, he eventually made a full recovery. We were extremely fortunate; I know many people reading this book are not so lucky.) I've found ACT enormously helpful in dealing with these difficult events in my own life, and I've also used it to help many others.

9

However, what's impressed me most of all with the ACT model is its universal applicability. Back in 2015 I wrote an ACT program for the World Health Organization, for use in refugee camps. The WHO have now used this program in a number of different countries, including Turkey, Uganda and Syria, to help refugees cope with multiple massive reality slaps: warfare, persecution, violence; deaths of loved ones; having to leave their homes, jobs and countries; and struggling to survive in the bleak living conditions of a refugee camp. I must confess, I was initially doubtful about the program; I wondered how it could possibly help people facing such great adversity. So I was both relieved and delighted when the WHO finally published their research several years later: the refugees not only liked the program, but found it very helpful for coping with their harsh life circumstances.

The book you're reading is very similar to the WHO program. I've divided it into three sections. Part 1 is titled 'Regroup', which means to reorganise yourself after a setback, and recollect your composure. Our main focus here is on how to take care of yourself, and deal with all those painful thoughts and feelings. Part 2 is titled 'Rebuild'. As the name suggests, here we look at how to rebuild your life, one small step at a time — no matter how extensive and severe the wreckage may be. Part 3 is titled 'Revitalise'. Here we look at how to bring back your vigour and vitality, and appreciate what life still has to offer. (Again, this may sound impossible right now.)

As a supplement to this book, I've created a free eBook called *The Reality Slap: Extra Bits*. As the name suggests, it contains additional resources — mostly free audio recordings of the exercises within this book. You can get the eBook from the 'Free Resources' page on my website, www.thehappinesstrap.com.

At this point, your mind may protest; it might insist that your case is different, this book won't help and your life will remain empty or unbearable. If so, rest assured: those are perfectly natural thoughts that many people have when they're new to this approach. And the fact is, even though this book is very likely to help you, I can't actually *guarantee* it. However, here's what I *can* guarantee: I guarantee that if you stop reading now, because your mind has doubts, then you definitely *won't* get any benefit from this book!

So if your mind is casting doubt, how about we just let it have its say? Let it tell you whatever it wants, but don't let that stop you from reading. Let your mind chatter away like a radio playing in the background, and together let's explore ... how to survive and thrive when life hits hard.

2

FIRST THINGS FIRST

Natalie's face was as pale as a winter moon. Tears streamed down her cheeks and splashed on her blouse, and her whole body shook as she cried. Ten days earlier, her teenage son had been struck and instantly killed by a hit-and-run driver. The police had still not managed to find the offender. 'My heart has broken into a million pieces,' said Natalie when she managed to get some words out amidst her sobbing. 'What can I do? What can I do?' she kept saying. 'I don't know what to do.'

Focus on what's in your control

When loss or trauma tears a gaping hole in our universe, most of us feel a daunting sense of powerlessness, as we struggle to come to terms with terrible events over which we have little or no control. So in this chapter, we're going to look at some basic practical tips to deal with the immediate aftermath of a reality slap.

The first step is to recognise that fear and anxiety are inevitable; they are normal, natural responses to life-disrupting situations infused with threat and uncertainty. And we easily start worrying about all sorts of things that are out of our control: what might happen in the future, and how this might affect us or our loved ones, and what will happen then, and so on. It's also easy to get lost in dwelling on the past: reliving those painful events, wondering what we could have done differently, imagining how that might have changed what happened, trying to figure out just who or what was to blame. The problem is, the more we focus on what's not in our control, the more hopeless, anxious or angry we're likely to feel. So the single most useful thing that anyone can do in response to any type of loss, crisis or trauma is to *focus on what's in your control*.

We can't control what happens in the future. We can't control what happened in the past. We can't control what other people do. And we definitely can't control our thoughts and feelings; there's no way to eliminate all those painful emotions and memories and somehow magically replace them with joy and happiness. But we *can* control what we *do* — here and now — with our arms and legs, our hands and our feet; we *can* control the physical actions we take. So this is where we need to focus our energy and our attention. This is the first step in surviving reality slaps: take control of your actions. Let's explore some of the ways we can do this.

No one is an island

When Shanti's husband left her and ran off with her childhood friend (with whom he'd been having an affair for two years), Shanti was, in her own words, 'shattered'. Her emotional storms included roaring floods of rage, torrential downpours of sadness, and gale force winds of anxiety, shame and embarrassment. Shanti reacted to her loss by hiding away from the outside world. She cut off contact from her friends and family, locked herself away inside her house. Michelle did something very similar, following a violent sexual assault. So did Dave, after he lost his job. Shanti, Michelle and Dave all had similar motivations for their isolation. They didn't want to see other people because they didn't want to talk about what had happened. They were afraid it would be too awkward, too uncomfortable; that it would bring up too many painful feelings and memories.

With Helen and Philip, the motivation for withdrawal was somewhat different. Helen's husband died suddenly and unexpectedly from a massive heart attack. Philip's husband died over several months from pancreatic carcinoma. Following these losses, Helen and Philip withdrew from friends and family mainly because they were exhausted; they just didn't have the energy to cope with social interaction.

Sometimes we may withdraw from specific groups of people. This is most likely when they still have something we have lost. When we see the huge discrepancy between their life and ours, it can be too painful to bear. For example, after her baby girl died from meningitis, Yoko withdrew from all her friends who had children; Alana did the same after her miscarriage. For both of them, it was just too painful to be around other families with young kids.

Rada's reality slap came in the form of a medical condition called fibromyalgia (or fibrositis). She had intense painful burning and throbbing sensations in her upper arms, shoulders, neck, back and abdomen, along with headaches, stiffness, extreme tiredness and fatigue. This severely limited her ability to do many of the daily activities she had previously taken for granted. So Rada withdrew from her loved ones because a) it was so exhausting for her to socialise, and b) it was so physically painful and tiring to get out of the house.

There are so many different reasons why we may retreat from those we are closest to. In some cases, we might not want to 'be a burden' to others; we don't wish to 'impose on them' or 'make them uncomfortable'. Or we may see that others are awkward and don't really know how to be with us or what to say to us — and, of course, that's uncomfortable for us as well as for them. Or we may get hooked by some stoic belief that 'I should be able to get through this on my own; I don't need anyone else'.

All of these reactions are completely normal and natural. (Yes, I know I've used that phrase quite a few times already in this book — but it's so important to keep repeating this message, because we are so quick to judge our own reactions as abnormal or defective or 'wrong'.) The problem is, when we withdraw from others it usually amplifies our suffering. You've probably heard the phrase 'humans are social animals'. If we wish to thrive, we need to spend quality time with others. Yet, all too often, when reality slaps us around we pull away from the people who care about us most. And, cocooned in our misery, cut off from loved ones, our pain only increases.

So it's important that we reach out to others — as long as they are caring, supportive and understanding. Who do you know that you can connect with? And how might you connect with them? Face to face? Phone calls? Video chats? Text message? Reaching out to others is something that's in our control. And keep in mind, it's fine to set time limits on how much time you spend together and what you do: 'Just called you to touch base; I can only chat for 5 minutes', 'Yes, sure — please do drop by, but probably 30 minutes is all I can cope with right now', 'If it's okay with you, I don't really want to talk about what happened', 'I don't want to talk, I just want you to hold me', 'Let's just watch a movie.'

It's also fine to say 'no'. If you're genuinely not up to being with others, honour that; decline the invitation. Likewise, if you are interacting with others and you feel like you need a break, it's absolutely fine to leave. Just let them know, 'I'm sorry, I need a break, I'm a bit overwhelmed right now.' Then go for a walk or retire to another room.

Unfortunately, one of the issues we often encounter is that other people don't have a clue how to treat us; they try to help, but all too often it falls flat. They may offer us platitudes — 'Everything happens for a reason' — or tell us to 'Be strong!' or try to push us into thinking 'positively' or 'rationally'. Or they may actively avoid asking us about what happened and how we're feeling, and try instead to distract us, change the topic. Or they may start talking about how things will be so much better in the future, or giving us advice on how to fix our problems, or getting preachy on us: 'God only gives us what we can handle.' And it's not their fault; they're usually trying their best to help and support — unfortunately, the society we live in doesn't teach any of us how to do this well.

Experiment

A quick Google search will reveal a vast electronic warehouse of advice on how to cope with your reality slap. And some of it's very good, and some of it's absolute rubbish — and absolutely nothing you find there will hold true for everyone. So we really need to experiment, to try different things and find out what works for us.

With that caution in mind, I will share two practical tips. First, a lot of people find it helpful to get out into the fresh air. Walks in nature are often quite comforting, because there's a sense of connection with something bigger, and the relief of escape from the challenges of life indoors. Out in nature it's easy to be yourself; you don't have to put on a brave face for the grass and the trees and the sky. You don't have to do anything at all. You can walk and breathe and notice the world around you, and let yourself feel whatever you're feeling.

Second, be wary of making big decisions. It's hard to make big decisions at the best of times — and it's doubly so following a reality slap, because we don't have all our mental faculties. We're often exhausted or sleep deprived; our minds are trying to grapple with so many different things that we find it hard to think straight. So if you do have big decisions to make, consider: would it be better to postpone them for a while, or delegate them to someone you trust? If those aren't options for you, at the very least use the 'dropping anchor' practice in Chapter 5 to ground and centre yourself before making that decision.

Many popular ideas about how to cope with grief, loss and trauma appeal to common sense but have no scientific validity. And one of these is the notion that you 'have to express your feelings'. Well, the fact is, you don't. For sure, *most* people find it's helpful to express their feelings — and if you think or know that this would be helpful for you, there are many ways to do it. The simplest way is to talk honestly and openly about what you're feeling, to your friends, family, a support group or a therapist. And a very popular alternative is to write about your feelings in a journal. However, if you're a creative type you might prefer to express your feelings in the form of poetry, prose, music, painting, drawing, sculpting, or even dance.

However, it's important to know that not everyone finds it helpful to do this; and it's definitely *not* essential! You can survive and thrive in the face of your reality slap without ever talking or writing about your feelings. So if you're not sure that expressing your feelings is for you, arguably the best option is to experiment with it and observe what happens. If you find it helpful, keep doing it; if not, stop.

A balancing act

The term 'self-care' might make you roll your eyeballs and groan loudly. But we do need to talk about it. Of course, right now, even the thought of 'self-care' may be overwhelming. And, if so, that's okay. Over the next few chapters you'll learn how to handle that sense of feeling overwhelmed and gently motivate yourself to do what's important.

Self-care is a bit of a balancing act. On the one hand, we want to give ourselves a break; take the pressure off ourselves; drop some of our responsibilities; take time to rest up and recuperate. On the other hand, we want to keep doing things that are healthy for ourselves. So for example, many of us will benefit from increased rest and 'downtime' following a reality slap; this makes sense because shocking life events eat up a lot of our energy; emotional storms are exhausting; and often, on top of all that, our sleep is disrupted. However, if we go to the extreme of staying in bed or lying on the couch for large parts of the day, for weeks upon end — well, that's likely to make us worse in the long term, not better.

Likewise, many people turn to comfort eating — chocolate, ice-cream, pizza — or drinking more alcohol than usual. In moderation, this isn't likely to be an issue; but if we do this excessively, it's going to create more problems on top of those we already have.

Same deal with exercise; it's normal that our exercise routines drop off, given the stress and strain of what we're going through. But if we give up on all exercise, then our health is going to suffer; it's so important to keep the body moving. This is especially so if you have a chronic illness or injury, like Rada. Because of all the pain, stiffness and exhaustion she experienced with her fibromyalgia, Rada simply couldn't do the physical activities she'd previously enjoyed for exercise and fitness, especially Latin dancing and aerobics. But without any physical exercise at all, fibromyalgia gets worse over time — so does almost any chronic illness you can think of, from diabetes to heart disease, from asthma to hypertension. This meant that Rada had to find new ways of exercising within the limitations imposed by her illness. Initially this involved basic stretching and strengthening exercises assigned by her physiotherapist, and extremely short walks assisted by a walking stick.

So it's worth spending a bit of time on creating a self-care plan. Take some time to consider how can you look after yourself physically through exercise, healthy eating, moderating any drug and alcohol use, appropriate rest and relaxation, and sensible sleep routines. At the same time, be realistic: if this all seems too hard — too much, too soon, too overwhelming — then it's okay to leave it for now. By the time you get to Chapter 18, 'Breaking bad habits', you'll have all the tools you need to effectively motivate yourself.

And don't forget about hobbies, sports, creative pursuits and other interests. These often fly out the window during times of upheaval. Sometimes it is wise to put these activities on the back burner for a while, as you focus on dealing with your problems. However, for many people, the sooner you can get back into these activities, the better. You might not initially enjoy them as much as you used to; you might be too emotional or tired or drained to engage in them fully. But if you persist, you may be surprised at how they comfort, encourage or sustain you amidst your suffering.

Obviously you need to adapt self-care so that it suits your unique circumstances. If you're recovering from major surgery, chemotherapy or a serious illness, you won't be able to work out in the gym; but there may be gentle exercises you can do while in bed. And once you're able to get out of bed, you can gradually build up your strength over time with simple exercises your doctor can recommend. If your reality slap doesn't involve injury or illness, you'll obviously have many more exercise options but you might not have the energy to do your usual routines, in which case, give yourself permission to do something easier, like going for a walk.

When Natalie kept repeating, 'What can I do?' she was asking a valuable question. There was nothing she could do to change the past, to bring her son back, to heal her fragmented heart. However, she was able to do tiny little acts of self-care — an important step in regaining a semblance of control over her life.

Remember: self-care doesn't have to involve great effort. Every time you brush your teeth, have a shower, eat something healthy, that's self-care. So is reaching out to friends, listening to music you love, or reading this book. And every little bit of self-care counts (even if your mind says it doesn't).

3

KIND WORDS

When reality slaps you hard and leaves you reeling, what do you want most from your closest friends and family? Most of us want pretty much the same thing. We want to know there is someone there for us: someone who truly cares about us; someone who takes the time to understand us; someone who recognises our pain and appreciates how badly we are suffering; someone who will make the time to be with us and allow us to share our true feelings without expecting us to cheer up or put on a brave face and pretend everything is okay; someone who will support us, treat us kindly and offer to help; someone who demonstrates through their actions that we are not alone. So here's the burning question: if we'd like others to treat us in this way — with caring, understanding and kindness — why do most of us treat ourselves so badly?

When reality slaps us around, we need all the kindness we can get. But for most of us, this isn't so easy to access. Why not? Because our minds have a natural tendency to judge us, criticise us, beat us up; to pull out a big stick and give us a hiding; to kick us when we're already down. Our minds may tell us we're not being strong enough, or we should be handling things better, or that others are far worse off than we are so we have nothing to complain about. They may tell us to get a grip, or sort ourselves out or stop being weak or pathetic. In some cases, our minds may even say that we are to blame for what happened.

For example, when someone we love dies, the mind might blame us for not having loved them enough, or not having been there enough, or not having told them enough how much we loved them; and sometimes even for not having prevented their death (especially common in cases of suicide)! One of my clients blamed himself for surviving a plane crash. His mind told him it was not fair that he had survived when twelve other passengers had died — that he 'didn't deserve to live'. (This is known as 'survivor guilt'.) Another client blamed herself for her son's schizophrenia: 'It was my fault; I gave him bad genes.'

Even if it doesn't launch into a personal attack, the mind is often callous, cold and uncaring; and, rather than help us cope, it crushes our spirit. It may tell us we can't cope, or that life's not worth living; or it may tell us to stop moaning, whining, complaining; or it may conjure up terrible fears about what's to come. And as I keep saying, all of this is normal — but it's not particularly helpful. So what's the alternative?

Hippy shit!

Antonio grimaced. A huge, muscle-bound Italian–Australian cop, he crossed his arms tightly across his chest. 'Don't give me that hippy shit!' he growled. Antonio's wife, Cathy, had pushed him to come and see me, and he sure wasn't trying to hide his resentment. Several weeks earlier, Antonio's baby girl, Sophia, had died from SIDS. Both he and Cathy were absolutely devastated, but they were both handling their grief very differently.

Cathy was doing many of the things we discussed in the last chapter: reaching out to friends and family, expressing her feelings, allowing herself to cry (sometimes for hours on end), and mostly taking good care of herself. In stark contrast, Antonio was cutting off from just about everyone and spending every evening in front of the TV, saying little but drinking heavily. And whenever Cathy tried to talk to him about their loss, their heartache, their suffering, Antonio would get angry and shut her down.

Despite his resentment at seeing me, Antonio cared deeply about Cathy and he wanted to make things better. He was quickly able to see that his behaviour was largely an attempt to escape pain. He loved his work, and during the day he could throw himself into the job, and mostly forget about his loss. But at home, it was a different story. Everything there reminded him of baby Sophia — most especially his wife. And with those reminders came pain like he'd never known. Drinking, refusing to talk, zoning out in front of the TV: these behaviours gave him some relief from that terrible pain — but at a huge cost to his relationship with his wife.

'I'm a fucking arsehole,' he said. 'I should be there for her — but I'm not. It's just, it's just … I just don't fucking want to think about it. It's too, it's just too … ah, I'm so fucking weak. I'm pathetic.'

'You're pretty good at beating yourself up,' I said.

'Yeah, well I fucking deserve it, don't I?'

'And is all that beating yourself up helping you to deal with the situation?'

'What do you think?' he asked with heavy sarcasm. 'Of course it fucking isn't.'

'So,' I said, 'given it's not really helping, are you open to trying something different?'

Antonio looked at me, suspiciously. 'Like what?'

'Like actually being kind to yourself.'

'Don't give me that hippy shit!' he growled.

Antonio's reaction was not uncommon. Many people initially resist the idea of self-kindness. 'What's hippyish about it?' I asked.

'I know what you're up to,' he said. 'Cathy's been banging on about this for days, this whatchaacallit — self-compassion. You're seriously gonna try and sell that shit to me?'

I took a deep breath. 'If I ask you a question, will you give me an honest answer?'

He shrugged. 'Sure.'

'Okay. So let's suppose you're travelling with a friend. And it's really tough. It's a dangerous journey and you're doing it hard, and all sorts of terrible things keep happening. It's knocking you around, and you're really struggling to keep going.'

Antonio shifted uncomfortably in his chair.

'Now,' I continued, 'as you carry on with the journey, what kind of friend do you want by your side? A friend who says, "Ah, shut up! Stop your whinging. I don't want to hear about it. Stop being such a wimp. Suck it up and get on with it, you big pussy!" … Or a friend who says, "This is really shit. But hey, we're in this together. I've got your back, and I'm with you every step of the way."'

Antonio cleared his throat. 'Well, obviously the second one,' he said.

'So what kind of friend are you being to yourself?' I asked. 'Are you more like the first or the second?'

What is self-compassion?

There are quite a few definitions of self-compassion floating around, and they all boil down to this: 'Acknowledge your pain, respond with kindness'. Doesn't sound like much, but those six words summarise a wealth of wisdom. Self-compassion means being real with yourself: recognising the fact that you're in pain, you're hurting; and then actively doing something kind, caring and supportive to help ease your suffering.

The bottom line is, if we can learn how to treat ourselves kindly we'll be much better off at handling our pain and dealing with all those problems life just dumped on us. Yet many people are initially somewhat dismissive of self-compassion. They may think it's flowery, airy-fairy, New Age, hippyish or touchy-feely. Some see it as psychobabble without any scientific validity. Others perceive it as a religious practice. Men may see it as 'effeminate' or 'unmanly'. And gender aside, quite a few people see it as 'weak', 'soft', or 'not really dealing with your problems'.

But none of these are valid criticisms. Yes, for sure, there are religious practices for self-compassion, and over the years its merits have often been touted by hippies and New Agers. But times change. Self-compassion is now firmly in the domain of Western science. Many respected scientists have researched the benefits of self-compassion (without any religious element to it) and found it to be helpful with a wide range of problems, from anxiety and depression to grief and trauma.

There's nothing weak or unmanly about being kind to a friend who's in great pain; so surely the same is true when we're kind to ourselves? And the research tells us that self-compassion is actually very helpful for dealing with our problems; it helps us regroup and recharge, so we have the motivation and energy to take effective action.

Sometimes people confuse self-compassion with 'self-pity'. 'What's the use of feeling sorry for yourself?' they ask. But they've missed the point. Self-pity is the very opposite of self-compassion; it's an excessive absorption in your own troubles, wallowing in them without doing anything practical to help yourself. That's a far cry from the brief self-compassion strategies you'll learn in this book, where you quickly acknowledge your pain (without pity, without wallowing) and do something practical to relieve it.

I've had quite a few clients who've opposed self-compassion on the grounds that, 'I don't have time for this; I have to take care of my family'. I ask them, 'Have you ever flown on an airplane? Remember that warning they always give you: always put your own oxygen mask on first before giving assistance to others? There's a good reason for that warning: if you don't get your mask on within about 30 seconds, you'll pass out; and then you'll be no use to anyone. So think of this as putting on your oxygen mask; it'll help you cope a whole lot better, so you can be there to take care of others. At times people think self-compassion means 'giving up' or 'not dealing with your problems' — but this is a huge misunderstanding. Actually, self-compassion helps to keep you going *instead of* giving up, and gives you the strength to actually deal with your problems.

Some people resist self-compassion because they think it's selfish or self-indulgent. But if your best friend was struggling, going through a really tough patch, wouldn't you be there to support them, help them get through it? And if they accepted your help and kindness, would you judge them as self-indulgent or selfish? Of course you wouldn't. So why the double standard? If your friend deserves kindness and caring in their time of need, so do you.

Now notice what your mind has to say about that. Is your mind in agreement? Or is it protesting: 'No, I don't deserve it!' If it's the latter, please rest assured: we've all got many different versions of the 'Not Good Enough' story, and this particular version — *I'm unworthy, I don't deserve kindness* — is extremely common. Later in the book, we'll learn how to deal with 'Not Good Enough' stories, but for now, can you please simply acknowledge it's there. Say to yourself something like, 'Okay, here's my mind beating me up, criticising me, telling me I don't deserve this.' And after that, let your mind say whatever it wants. Don't debate or argue with it, because you almost certainly won't win. Just let your mind 'do its schtick' while you do the exercises that follow.

Acknowledging your pain

'Okay, I get your point,' said Antonio. 'But I don't think I can do that sort of stuff. As a cop, you learn to suck it up, get on with it.'

I nodded. 'Yes, your default setting is to be like the first friend: *"Suck it up, get on with it, stop whining, no one cares!"*'

Antonio nodded. 'That's pretty much it.'

'But if your best mate's daughter had just died, that's not what you'd say to him, is it?'

'No, of course not!'

'What would you say to him?'

'Ah, Jesus! I wouldn't have a fucking clue!'

'Well, just take a moment to think about it. Usually when people are in great pain, they want to hear two things: one, "I can see you're hurting"; two, "I'm here for you". So how would you say that in your own words?'

Antonio thought for a moment, then said, very softly, 'I guess I'd say, "This is really fucking shit, mate. It's the worst thing ever. It shouldn't happen to anyone. Especially not you. I'm here for ya …

whatever you need" ...' At this point his voice cracked. The 'tough cop' mask disappeared, and tears welled in his eyes.

Like many of us, Antonio knew how to be compassionate to others but struggled with applying this to himself. If you don't relate to that struggle — if you find it natural and easy to be kind and supportive to yourself — you're very lucky. I'm going to assume that most readers, like myself when I was first introduced to the concept, will find self-compassion quite challenging, so I'm going to introduce it in small steps. And the very first step is simply to acknowledge our pain. Because the fact is, reality slaps hurt. They hurt *so much*. And we so badly want that pain to stop — but all too often, it doesn't.

Kind self-talk has two main elements, both of which you can see in Antonio's speech:

1. acknowledge your pain
2. respond with kindness.

The first step

Acknowledging our pain simply means being honest with ourselves about just how much this hurts — without dwelling on it or wallowing in it or turning it into self-pity. So, for example, we wouldn't go into a long internal monologue: *This is awful. I can't bear it any longer. I've never felt so bad. When's it going to stop?* That's a recipe for misery and despair. We want to acknowledge our pain in a kind, honest way — just as we'd acknowledge the pain of a friend who was suffering.

One way to do this is to create a phrase that is short and easy to remember, that also helps us step back a little from our suffering — rather than falling into it. Terms such as 'Here is ...', 'I'm noticing ...',

'I'm having …' are particularly useful: 'Here is sadness', 'I'm noticing anger', 'I'm having feelings of despair'. This is an odd way of speaking — and that's deliberate. You see, in everyday language, we say things like, 'I am sad' or 'I am lonely' or 'I am angry' — and that makes it seem as if *I am the emotion*. But when we say things like 'I'm noticing sadness' or 'Here is loneliness' or 'I'm having feelings of anger', it helps us to step back a little, and see that these difficult feelings are not *who we are*; rather, they are experiences, passing through us.

These unusual ways of speaking — 'I'm noticing fear' or 'Here is anxiety' — usually help us to stand slightly back from our pain, to detach from it a little, which makes it less likely to sweep us away. And if you can't pinpoint the exact feeling you're noticing, or if there are so many you can't distinguish them, you can use terms like 'suffering', 'grief', 'hurt', 'loss', 'pain', or 'heartbreak': 'Here is suffering', 'I'm noticing heartbreak'. On the other hand, if your freeze response kicked in and cut off your feelings, you might say 'I'm noticing numbness', or 'Here is a feeling of emptiness'.

Another thing that can help is to include terms such as 'here and now' or 'in this moment'. If we say, 'Here and now, I'm noticing loss' or 'In this moment, grief is here' or 'Right here and now, I'm noticing anger', this helps us to remember the transient nature of painful thoughts and feelings — the way that, just like the weather, they continually change. Even during the worst days of your life, your emotions will change; at times you'll feel better and at times you'll feel worse. So 'here and now' you might be noticing sadness — but later you'll be noticing something else. Other terms you could use include 'this is an instant of', 'this is a moment of' or 'this is an experience of'. For example, 'This is a moment of great sadness' or 'This is an instant of anger'.

The idea is to play around with these words and come up with a phrase that works for you. Kristin Neff, the world's top researcher on self-compassion, likes to say, 'This is a moment of suffering'. There's something poetic in this phrase that appeals to many people. However, some people prefer everyday language. For example, Rada — who was suffering from fibromyalgia — preferred to say, 'This really hurts'. And remember Natalie, whose son died because of a hit-and-run? She came up with: 'I'm noticing heartbreak'. As for Antonio, he preferred the simple phrase, 'Here is …': 'Here is sadness', 'Here is anger' and so on. (One of my clients, after reading the first edition of this book, chose the phrase, 'This is a reality slap — and it hurts!').

I encourage you to try this right now.

Take a moment to notice any difficult feelings that are present right now, and label them: anger, sadness, anxiety, loneliness, etc.

And then, very slowly, using a calm, kind, peaceful inner voice, acknowledge it: 'I'm noticing …' or 'Here is …'.

Now, pause for a moment, and take a slow and gentle breath, in and out.

And now, try this once more.

Very slowly, in a calm, kind, peaceful inner voice, acknowledge: 'I'm noticing …' or 'Here is …'.

The second step, and bringing them both together

The next step, after we acknowledge our pain, is to remind ourselves to respond with kindness. So, for example, we might silently say things like, 'Be kind to yourself', 'Go easy on yourself', 'Give yourself a break', 'Ease off' or 'Gently does it'. Some people prefer to use a single word, like 'Gentle' or 'Kind'. Kristin Neff, the brilliant self-compassion researcher I mentioned above, says, 'May I be kind to myself'. Rada preferred to simply say, 'Be kind'. Natalie chose 'May I treat myself kindly'. Antonio, after quite a bit of struggle, chose 'Go easy on yourself'.

The idea is then to put both these steps — acknowledging your pain and responding with kindness — into a catchphrase you can use over and over:

'This really hurts. Be kind.'

'I'm noticing heartbreak. May I treat myself kindly.'

'Here is sadness. Go easy on yourself.'

'This is a moment of suffering. May I be kind to myself.'

Once you've done this, the aim is to repeat these words to yourself, using a calm, kind, peaceful inner voice (i.e. not one that is harsh, uncaring, demanding or bossy in tone) whenever you're struggling with your pain. This isn't a way to make your pain go away; the aim is to give you a sense of comfort and support, as if there's a caring friend by your side.

Also, keep in mind, this isn't a 'positive thinking' practice; you're not trying to get rid of 'negative' thoughts and replace them with 'positive' ones. If you try using self-compassion for that purpose, you'll soon be disappointed. Harsh, unhelpful or self-judgmental thoughts will continue to arise (later in the book, we'll discuss why this is). The aim here is to allow your thoughts and feelings to be as they are in this moment, while simultaneously bringing in some kind self-talk. In other words, rather than trying to get rid of unwanted thoughts, you're acknowledging they are present, allowing them to stay, and adding in some new ones to keep them company. (If this seems odd, it will make a lot more sense after you've read the next two chapters.)

In a moment, I'm going to ask you to try this out: create your own catchphrase, or pick one of the four I listed above, and say it to yourself with genuine kindness — using a calm, soft, gentle inner voice. (If you say it with a harsh, bossy or uncaring inner voice, it won't have the desired effect.)

But first, let me make a prediction. About 95 per cent of readers will do the exercise that follows and get some immediate benefit. About 5 per cent of readers will have a negative reaction; either nothing much at all will happen and you will be disappointed, or the exercise will bring up some difficult thoughts and feelings (most likely anxiety, self-criticism or some version of 'I don't deserve it'). If you're in the 5 per cent, rest assured — that's not a problem, because over the next few chapters, you'll learn a number of different skills that will make this a whole lot easier. Okay, enough of the preamble ... let's try it out.

Some kind words

I invite you now to find a comfortable position in which you are centered and alert. For example, if you're seated in a chair you could lean slightly forwards, straighten your back, drop your shoulders and press your feet gently onto the floor.

Now bring to mind whatever you are struggling with. Take a few moments to reflect on what has happened, and how it is affecting you. And notice what difficult thoughts and feelings arise.

Then using a kind and calm inner voice, speaking to yourself slowly and softly, take a moment to genuinely acknowledge your pain and respond with kindness. If you're stuck for ideas, try these words: 'This really hurts. Be kind.'

Now pause for a moment, and notice what happens.

And if you feel like it, take a breath — and ever so slowly and gently, allow the air to flow in and out of your lungs.

Then, once again, repeat this phrase with kindness.

Then pause for a moment, and notice what happens.

And again, if you feel like it, take a breath: breathing in and out, slowly and gently.

Now, one last time, repeat those kind words to yourself, infusing them with warmth, care and comfort.

And again, pause for a moment, and notice what happens.

So what happened? If nothing much happened, or it brought up difficult thoughts and feelings — that's not a problem; I'm confident this will change as you work through the book. For now, just acknowledge that at this point in time, this type of kind self-talk is not working for you. The good news is, there are many other ways to treat yourself kindly. For example, consider those acts of self-care we discussed last chapter. If you do these things on autopilot, or out of a sense of compliance, because your mind says 'You have to do this; you have to take care of yourself', they're still useful but they're unlikely to give you that sense of being kind to yourself. However, you can change that. The idea is to keep doing them — but see if, as you do them, you can 'sprinkle on' a sense of genuine warmth and caring. (You may not be able to do this — but have a go, anyway.) Likewise, in the next few chapters you'll learn a number of different skills for handling your pain differently, taking the impact out of it; and each time you apply these skills to ease your suffering, that's an act of kindness in itself.

On the other hand, maybe this exercise *did* help you tap into a sense of self-kindness. And even if you only had the tiniest glimmer of it, that's a good start; self-compassion is a skill, and like any skill it gets better with practice. So if this did happen for you, please play around with your kind self-talk. Keep playing with words until you find a phrase that resonates with you; then repeat it to yourself throughout the day — especially in those moments when life hurts most. And notice what it's like when you turn towards yourself with genuine kindness; appreciate that sense of befriending yourself. When reality slaps you hard, self-kindness is your greatest ally.

4

DROP THE STRUGGLE

Shanti could barely look at me. Her voice was quiet and drenched with despair. 'I just want to stop feeling this way!' she said. You may recall Shanti from Chapter 2. Her husband, Ravi, had been having an affair with Shanti's best friend for over two years. When Shanti found about it, Ravi left her and ran off with her friend, to start a new life in another city. Shame, anger, betrayal, injustice, loneliness, sadness and anxiety; all of this and more kept showing up. Of course Shanti wanted to 'stop feeling this way'. None of us like pain; we all want it gone. But how much control do we really have over our feelings?

As infants, toddlers and young children, we are largely controlled by our emotions. Fear, anger, sadness, guilt, frustration and anxiety: these emotions, and many others, push children around as if they are remote-controlled robots. If anger shows up, they shout or yell or lash out, or stomp their feet. If fear shows up, they hide or cry or run away. If sadness or disappointment show up, they sulk or cry or bawl.

Fortunately, as adults we are much less controlled by our feelings, and this is a good thing. We would all be in big trouble if our feelings controlled us. Imagine if you were at the mercy of your fear, anger, sadness and guilt; if it pushed you around exactly as it did when you were a child. How difficult would life be for you?

Of course, at times we all get pushed around by our emotions. We may lose our temper, get carried away by our fears, find ourselves overwhelmed with sadness, get crushed with guilt, or go into a fit of blind rage. But fortunately, this happens much less than it did in childhood (at least, for most people). And this is because, as we grew older, we learned all sorts of ways to control our feelings.

For example, we learned how to distract ourselves from unpleasant emotions via food, music, TV, books or games. And as we grew older, the number of potential distractions multiplied: exercise, work, study, hobbies, religion, computer games, email, gambling, sex, pornography, music, sport, drugs, alcohol, gardening, walking the dog, cooking, dancing and so on.

We also learned how to escape unpleasant feelings by avoiding the situations where they were most likely to occur; in other words, we learned to withdraw or stay away from the people, places, activities or tasks we found difficult or challenging.

Then there are all those thinking strategies we developed that, at times, could give us some relief from emotional pain. Most of us have a wealth of these strategies, such as:

- constructive problem-solving
- writing lists
- looking at the situation from a different perspective
- blaming or criticising others
- challenging negative thoughts
- positive thinking

- vigorously defending your position
- positive affirmations
- telling yourself inspirational quotes like, 'This too shall pass' or 'What does not hurt me makes me stronger'
- trivialising the issue or pretending it's not important, or joking about it
- comparing yourself to others who are worse off.

And, last but not least, we have all discovered that putting substances into our bodies — whether it be chocolate, ice-cream, pizza, sugar, tea, coffee, aspirin, paracetamol, alcohol, tobacco, recreational drugs, herbal remedies or prescription medication — often gives short-term relief from painful feelings.

And yet, even with all these clever ways to control our feelings, we continue to suffer psychologically. We are not free from emotional pain for long. Think of the happiest day of your life; how long did those joyous, happy feelings last before some anxiety, frustration, disappointment or irritation showed up? Not long, right? And that's on the happiest day of your life! So when reality slaps us around, most of these 'emotion control strategies' fail miserably.

The fact is that to live a full human life is to experience the full range of human emotions — not just the ones that 'feel good'. Our feelings are like the weather, continually changing: at times very pleasant, at other times extremely uncomfortable. And what would happen if we went through life believing, 'We should have good weather every day. There must be something seriously wrong if it's cold and wet outside'? If this was our attitude, how much would we struggle with reality? How much would our life shrink if we believed, 'I can't do the things that really matter to me, or be the person I want to be, unless the weather is good'?

When we talk about the weather this way it seems ridiculous. We know we can't control the weather, so we don't even try to. We let the weather do what it does and we change our clothes to adapt. But when it comes to emotions, most of us do the opposite — we try as hard as we can to get control of them! And this is quite natural; after all, everyone wants to feel good, and no one wants to feel bad. So we try to push our unwanted feelings away with quick fixes such as those mentioned above. And, of course, most of those things do reduce pain quite well at times — but for how long? How long do those feelings go away for, before they come back again? A few minutes? Perhaps a few hours if you're lucky?

As we journey through life, we all experience intense and uncomfortable emotions that we can't simply turn off at the flick of a switch. And you've undoubtedly discovered that often the strategies we use to control our emotions tend to impair our quality of life in the long term. This is most obvious when it comes to things such as drugs, alcohol, tobacco, chocolate and gambling — but if you look closely, with an open mind, you'll find it applies to any 'emotion control strategy' that we use *excessively* or *rigidly*.

Even something as healthy as exercise will become problematic if we use it *excessively* or *rigidly* to try to control our feelings. For example, some people suffering from anorexia exercise vigorously every day and, in the short term, this helps them to control their feelings of anxiety — to push away all those fears about getting fat — but, in the long term, it keeps their bodies in a state of extremely unhealthy thinness. This is obviously very different from exercising *flexibly*, to look after your health and wellbeing *wisely*.

Often, the disappointments and setbacks we encounter when we attempt to control our emotions just spur us on to try even harder, to find even cleverer ways to control how we feel. The hope is that one day we will find the ultimate strategy, one that will give us excellent control of our feelings. But, sooner or later, we realise this is a lost cause. To emphasise this point, whenever I give workshops or lectures, I ask all the parents in the room to raise their hands. Usually, this is about three-quarters of the audience. I say, 'Having a child enriches your life enormously and gives you some of the most wonderful feelings you will ever have — love, joy and tenderness, the likes of which you could never have imagined. But are those the only feelings they give you?'

Everyone shakes their heads and says, 'Nooooo!'

'What other feelings do children give you?' I ask.

There is a cacophony of responses: fear, anger, exhaustion, worry, guilt, sadness, pain, frustration, rejection, boredom and rage, to name but a few.

And there you have it: the things that make life rich and meaningful give rise to a wide range of feelings, both pleasant *and* painful. (This, of course, holds true for every loving relationship, not just those with our children. No wonder the philosopher Jean-Paul Sartre said, 'Hell is other people'.)

Unfortunately, this realisation can take a long time to come. It may take us a hundred self-help books, or twenty years of therapy, or five different types of prescription medication, or a dozen self-empowerment courses, or decades of silent struggle, or a lifetime of seeking advice from various 'experts' before we truly realise the simple truth: when it comes to painful emotions, we have not been well educated by our society. We have grown up learning only two ways of responding:

control or be controlled. And if these are our only two options, we will always be struggling.

Sometimes I have clients who react quite negatively to these ideas; they were clinging to the idea that recovering from their reality slap means no more painful thoughts and feelings. *If only!* As we recover from our losses and heal our wounds, those difficult thoughts, feelings and memories don't disappear. What happens is, we find a new way of responding to them. We learn how to handle them differently; how to take the impact out of them, so that when they arise, they can't hold us back from engaging in life. We learn how to access a centre of stillness, in the midst of our pain; how to 'create a space' within ourselves through which our feelings can freely flow — without pushing us around or bringing us down. I call this 'dropping the struggle'.

Struggle is exhausting

When we only have two options for responding to difficult thoughts and feelings — either 'control' or 'be controlled' — life becomes exhausting, because we invest so much time and energy in this futile struggle with our inner world. But there's a third way of responding to these difficult inner experiences; and it's so radically different to the other two ways, it often takes a while to understand it. So, to get a sense of what it involves, I invite you to do …

A simple three-step experiment

There are three steps to this experiment, and you will get much more out of it if you actually *do* it, rather than simply reading about it. It's very important, because it paves the way for the skills we're going to learn in the next chapter.

Step 1: Imagine that in front of you is everything that's important; both the pleasant things — like the people, movies, music, food, books and activities you love — and the unpleasant things — like all the challenges and problems you have to deal with. And imagine the book in your hands is made up of all the difficult thoughts, feelings, emotions, sensations, urges and memories that you find most difficult. (Take a few moments to name them.)

Step 2: *(Please don't do this next step if you have neck or shoulder or upper arm problems; instead, just vividly imagine what it would be like to do it.)* When you reach the end of this paragraph, take the book in both hands, grip it tightly around the edges, and hold it as far away from you as you possibly can. Push your arms out as far as you possibly can (without actually dislocating your shoulders!); straighten them fully at the elbows, and keep the book at arm's length. Hold it like that for about 1 minute and notice what the experience is like.

Did you find that uncomfortable or tiring? Imagine doing this all day long; how exhausting would it be? And imagine watching your favourite movie or TV show, or having a conversation, or eating a meal, or making love at the same time as doing this exercise. How much would it distract you or interfere with your enjoyment? This is what it is like when we try to control our emotions: we exert a huge amount of energy into pushing them away. Not only is this draining and distracting; it also pulls us out of the here-and-now and into an internal struggle. When we are trying hard to control our emotions, it is very difficult to be present and respond effectively to life's challenges. Now let's try something different.

Step 3: When you reach the end of this paragraph (again pretending this book is your thoughts and feelings), again push the book away from you, as hard as you can, for about 30 to 60 seconds. Then stop pushing, and instead, place the book gently on your lap, and let it sit there. And notice the difference this makes. And as you let it sit there, stretch your arms, take a breath, and with a sense of genuine curiosity, scan your surroundings, and notice what you can see and hear around you.

Did you notice how letting the book sit on your lap was so much easier, so much less distracting and so much less effort than getting caught up in it or keeping it at arm's length? Did you notice that when you disentangled yourself from it, stopped struggling with it and made space for it, you could be fully present with the world around you?

This is a radically different way of responding to painful inner experiences. I call it 'dropping the struggle'. This means opening up and making room for our thoughts, feelings and memories; letting them come and stay and go in their own good time. We're not letting them push us around or sweep us away; and nor are we investing our energy in trying to fight with or run from them.

When I took Shanti through this exercise, she said, 'Yes, but this is just a book. I can't do that with real feelings.' And she was right. It's easy to rest a book on your lap; a whole lot harder to do something similar with actual thoughts and feelings. So let's now have a crack at the real thing.

5

WHEN STORMS ARISE

With great loss comes great pain. Often there is sadness and sorrow. And often there is guilt or regret. (This is especially likely if we somehow contributed to the events that happened — or, at least, believe we did.) In addition, there is usually a lot of anger and fear. This is because all major losses pose a threat to us. They may threaten our way of life, our security, our physical health, our mental health, our wellbeing, our loved ones, or many other things we hold precious. And as we discussed in Chapter 1, when we encounter a significant threat we immediately go into 'fight-or-flight' mode. But if fight or flight seems futile, the 'freeze' response kicks in. In humans, the 'fight' response fosters anger, irritation, resentment or rage; while the 'flight' response fosters fear, anxiety, insecurity or panic. In contrast, the 'freeze' response give rise to numbness, lethargy, apathy and fatigue.

And as if all of that's not enough, our minds then start pouring fuel onto the fire. They generate all sorts of anxious, angry, judgmental or hopeless thoughts, and often dredge up painful memories too. We easily get hooked by these thoughts and pulled into worrying about the future, dwelling on the past, blaming ourselves or others, or obsessing about things that are out of our control.

These are all normal responses to challenging situations awash with instability and uncertainty, so we expect them to happen repeatedly after a reality slap. We can think of these reactions as 'emotional storms': difficult thoughts blow wildly around inside our head, while intense feelings and emotions whip through our body. And when an emotional storm sweeps us away, there's nothing effective we can do to deal with the difficult challenges life has placed in front of us.

So how do we handle emotional storms? Well, in real life, when a storm blows up the boats in the harbour all drop anchor. Why? Because if they don't, they'll get damaged or swept out to sea. And of course, when a boat drops anchor, that doesn't magically make the storm go away — anchors can't control the weather. But it does hold the boat steady until the storm passes. So we're going to do something very similar — we're going to learn how to 'drop anchor' when emotional storms blow up inside us.

The ACE formula: Acknowledge, Connect, Engage

Anchor-dropping exercises can be as short as 10 seconds or as long as 10 minutes, and you can do them any time, any place — no matter what you're feeling. There are literally hundreds of different ways to drop anchor (and you can easily invent new ones of your own) but they all revolve around the simple 'ACE' formula:

A: **acknowledge** your thoughts and feelings

C: **connect** with your body

E: **engage** in what you're doing.

So let's go through this right now. You can do this exercise no matter how you're feeling right now — happy or sad, anxious or angry, neutral or numb.

The ACE formula in practice

A: Acknowledge your thoughts and feelings

Silently and kindly acknowledge whatever is 'showing up' inside you: thoughts, feelings, emotions, memories, sensation, urges. Take the stance of a curious child, who's never encountered something of this nature before. With openness and curiosity, notice what's going on in your inner world.

Quickly scan your body for feelings and sensations, and note what kind of thoughts are passing through your head. As you do this, often it's helpful to describe what's 'showing up' inside you, with phrases like 'I'm noticing' or 'I'm having'. (Yes, the same phrases we discussed in Chapter 3.) For example, you might silently say to yourself something like, 'I'm noticing anxiety', or 'I'm having a feeling of sadness' or 'I'm noticing numbness' or 'I'm having scary thoughts' or 'I'm noticing my mind obsessing' or 'I'm having thoughts about being a bad person'.

The idea here is to acknowledge your thoughts and feelings without judging them, fighting them, or trying to get rid of them. You're simply acknowledging that right now, in this moment, they are here.

And while continuing to acknowledge your thoughts and feelings, also ...

C: Connect with your body

Come back into and connect with your physical body. Find your own way of doing this. You could try some or all of the following, or experiment with your own methods:

- Slowly push your feet into the floor.

- Slowly straighten your back and your spine.

- Slowly press your fingertips together.

- Slowly stretch your arms or your neck or shrug your shoulders.

If chronic illness or an injury limits what you can do with your physical body, you can adapt this exercise to accommodate it. Because of her fibromyalgia and the intense, painful sensations she experienced in her upper body, Rada didn't want to do most of the things above. She was okay with pushing her feet down into the floor, but not the other suggestions, so between us we came up with these alternatives:

- Slowly and gently, breathe in and out.

- Slowly and gently, adjust your position in the chair to one more comfortable.

- Slowly and gently, move your eyes from side to side.

- Slowly and gently, raise your eyebrows then lower them.

In other words, be creative; anything that helps you connect with your body in some way will suffice. As you do this practice, you are not trying to escape, avoid or distract yourself from what is happening in your inner world. Nor are you trying to get rid of those difficult thoughts and feelings. (Remember: anchors don't make storms go away.) The aim is to remain aware of your thoughts and feelings, continue to acknowledge their presence ... and at the same time, connect with your body and actively move it. Why? So you can gain a lot more control over your physical actions; over what you do with your arms, hands, legs and feet, face and mouth. Trying to control your thoughts and feelings often fails or creates new problems. But taking control of your actions is a different story; it will enable you to act effectively as the storm continues to rage.

Now as you **acknowledge** your thoughts and feelings, and **connect** with your body, also ...

E: Engage in what you're doing

Get a sense of where you are and refocus your attention on the activity you are doing. Again, find your own way of doing this. You could try some or all of the following suggestions, or find your own methods:

- Look around the room and notice five things you can see.

- Notice three or four things you can hear.

- Notice what you can smell or taste, or sense inside your nose or mouth.

- Notice what you are doing.

End the exercise by giving your full attention to the activity you're doing.

The idea is to run through this ACE cycle slowly three or four times, to turn it into a 2 to 3 minute exercise.

To help you get the hang of this, I've created some free audio recordings of 'dropping anchor' exercises, varying from 1 minute to 11 minutes in length. You can download them from links in my free eBook, *The Reality Slap: Extra Bits*, which you'll find on the 'Free resources' page on www.thehappinesstrap.com.

Anchors don't control storms

Sometimes when I take people through this exercise, they complain, 'It isn't working!' So I ask, 'What do you mean, it's not working?' They usually reply with something like, 'I don't feel any better. It's not making these feelings go away'. So I explain that, just as anchors don't control storms, this isn't a way to control your feelings.

The aims of dropping anchor are:

- to gain more control of our physical actions — so we can act more effectively when difficult thoughts and feelings are showing up

- to reduce the impact and influence of our thoughts and feelings; when we're consciously aware of our thoughts and feelings, they lose their control over us — whereas when we're on autopilot they easily jerk us around like a puppet on a string

- to interrupt worrying, rumination, obsessing or the many other ways we get lost inside our heads

- to interrupt problematic behaviours, such as fighting and arguing with loved ones, or withdrawing and hiding away from them, or inappropriately using drugs and alcohol

- to help us refocus and engage in the activity we are doing, when our thoughts and feelings keep pulling us out of it.

There are other benefits to this practice, which we'll explore later, but there's one thing I'd like to clarify straight away: *you're not trying to distract yourself* from these difficult thoughts and feelings.

Remember: A is for acknowledge. When we keep acknowledging the thoughts, feelings, emotions, sensation urges and memories that are present, that's the very opposite of distraction. If we start trying to distract ourselves from these inner experiences — get away from them, try to ignore them, pretend that they aren't there — we're right back into the struggle we discussed last chapter: 'control or be controlled'. Distraction's not wrong or bad — but you already know how to do it, and you know it only gives short-term relief. Our aim here is to do something radically different: to step out of that struggle; to let our thoughts and feelings be as they are; to let them come and go in their own good time. Think again of that boat dropping anchor in the harbour — it's not trying to get rid of the storm, or distract from it. Dropping anchor holds the boat steady while the storm comes and goes in its own good time.

So if you are in intense emotional pain — for example, if the person you love is dying, or you're flooded with panic, or struggling with crushing loneliness — it's highly unlikely that your pain will disappear as you drop anchor. But what you can expect is that it'll lose some of its impact; you'll drain away its power so it can't jerk you around as much. And if you practise for several minutes you'll often start to experience a sense of calmness, even as your inner storm continues.

On the other hand, if you're just feeling a little bit sad or anxious, then as you drop anchor the pain will quite often reduce, or even disappear. And of course, you can enjoy that when it happens — but keep in mind that's a bonus, not the main aim. If you start using these techniques to try to avoid, escape, get rid of or distract from painful thoughts and feelings, you'll soon be frustrated and complain that 'It's not working'.

The first time I took Shanti through this exercise, we spent a good 5 minutes on it, cycling several times through A-C-E. Her transformation was profound. Her posture changed from hunched over to upright; her voice become stronger and more lively; her facial expression changed from despairing to peaceful; instead of staring at the floor, she was looking right at me. I said to her, 'You know those moments where the clouds part, and the sunlight comes shining through? That's what this is like for me. Five minutes ago, you were so lost in all those thick black clouds of thoughts and feelings, it was like you'd disappeared from the room; but now, you're back.' A warm smile played across her face. Shanti's thoughts and feelings hadn't disappeared (anchors don't make storms go away), but they had lost a lot of their impact, and now she could fully engage in our session.

Back to the present

One aim of the anchor-dropping exercise is to train up your ability to focus on and engage in what you're doing. Many of us find this challenging at the best of times, but it's exceptionally hard to do this after reality slaps. Have you found it hard to be fully present with your loved ones? Does your attention keep wandering? Do you keep 'zoning out' or 'drifting off'? Are you 'only half-present' or 'absent-minded'? Are you doing things on autopilot, or 'just going through the motions'? Do you easily lose track of what you're doing? Do you do things poorly that you'd normally do a lot better because you aren't focused on the task? Do you find events and activities less pleasurable or satisfying than they used to be, because you can't really engage in them fully?

Even when life is normal, it's often hard for us to focus, engage and be present. But when reality slaps us around, most of us find that disengagement and distractibility rise to whole new levels. And again, our fight, flight or freeze responses play a big role in this. Let's start with fight-or-flight mode. When our ancient ancestors were out hunting wild animals, that was a dangerous activity. And the further they got from the safe and familiar territory they called home, the greater the level of threat. So if you're out late at night on a hunting mission, you don't want to be staring peacefully into a campfire for long periods of time; you want to be getting up regularly, looking around for wolves, bears and rival clans. Fight-or-flight mode encourages this; it predisposes you to keep shifting your attention — which therefore makes it hard to focus or concentrate. What about freeze mode? Well, here your nervous system wants you to lie still and be quiet until the threat has gone — so it helps you to 'zone out', 'drift off', take your attention away from what's going on. During the worst parts of your reality slap, this helps you escape the horror to some extent; but in the weeks or months that follow the same response keeps activating, which again makes it hard to engage in or focus on what you're doing. So my hope is that you'll transfer the basic principles of dropping anchor to everyday life: wherever you are, whatever you're doing, see if you can catch yourself drifting off or zoning out, gently acknowledge it, and then refocus on the activity at hand.

One way our minds pull us out of the present is by dragging us back into the past. One of my clients, Ali, was an Iraqi refugee. He had been horribly tortured under Saddam Hussein's regime. He had dared to publicly criticise the government so they threw him into prison for several months. During that time, his jailers did the most horrific things to his body. Two years later, as he sat on the other side of my office, Ali kept having 'flashbacks' to those events. A flashback is a memory that is so vivid and incredibly real, it's as if it is actually happening here and now. If you've never had one, you can scarcely imagine how terrifying it can be.

Whenever Ali tried to talk to me about his time in prison, a flashback would hijack him; his body would go rigid, his eyes would glaze over and his face would go pale. Dragged back into the past, he would relive the torture as if it were happening again. So my first task, before addressing any of his other serious problems, was to teach him how to get himself back to the present.

I asked him to practise dropping anchor at least twenty to thirty times a day. That may seem like a lot, but he was suffering from PTSD (post-traumatic stress disorder) and I knew those flashbacks would repeatedly hijack him, pouncing on him unexpectedly and carrying him off to the past to relive his nightmares. So I wanted him to become an expert at returning to the here and now. And I strongly encourage you to do the same.

After any significant loss, painful memories tend to show up repeatedly: about the events that happened or what led up to them, or what life was like before the slap. When we are grieving, even the most beautiful memories can trigger great pain. As we remember all those good times when we were with the person who died (or the person we broke up with), or doing the job we loved, or doing all those activities we could enjoy before injury or illness made them impossible, all sorts of painful emotions tend to show up. Later in the book we'll look at ways to work with and handle these memories, but for now, the aim is simply to drop anchor.

So when a painful memory shows up, begin with A: acknowledge your thoughts and feelings. Say to yourself, 'I'm noticing a memory' or 'Here's a painful memory' or 'I'm having a memory'. If possible, it's better to specifically label the memory — for example, 'Here's a memory of my mother', 'I'm having a memory of the funeral', 'I'm noticing a memory of the car crash'. Acknowledge the memory and all the painful feelings that go with it, then connect with your body and engage in what you're doing.

Antonio found this practice very helpful. He had deeply distressing memories of finding baby Sophia in her crib — unmoving, silent and blue. Whenever they resurfaced, he'd drop anchor and say to himself, 'Here is a memory of Sophia.' Often, he'd add, 'This really hurts. Go easy on yourself.' He wouldn't try to push it away or distract himself; he'd acknowledge it and allow it to be there — and at the same time, he'd connect with his body through stretching, and then engage with the world. Over time, this practice made a big difference; the memories still hurt when they resurfaced, but they lost a lot of their impact.

Any time, any place

We can do an anchor-dropping exercise any time and any place, and it instantly brings us back into the present so we can engage in life and focus on the task at hand. We don't want to wait until 'emotional storms' blow up; the idea is to practise these exercises throughout the day. We can practise in those many moments when we 'drift off' into our thoughts and feelings; at red traffic lights, or during ad breaks on the TV, or waiting in a queue, or at our desk before starting work, or in our lunchbreak, or first thing when we get out of bed. We can practise at times when our emotional weather is mild; when we're just a little bit grumpy or down or worried. We can practise when we're bored or impatient — instead of turning to our smartphones for distraction. We can practise with any inner experience — thoughts, images, memories, emotions, feelings, sensations, urges, impulses — in any combination.

As with any exercise in this book, there are all sorts of ways you can modify dropping anchor. For instance, when it comes to C — connect with your body — you might choose to stand up and give your body a stretch, and hold that stretch and feel your muscles lengthen. Or you could push your palms and fingers against each other and feel the muscles contract in your neck, arms and shoulders. Or you could press your hands down on the arms of your chair. Or firmly massage the back of your neck and scalp. Or breathe in and out, slowly and gently. Or ever so slowly adjust your position in the chair, and notice what your body does to enable that. Or slowly look around the room and notice how you're using your neck, head and eyes. Or, if you know how to do them and you're somewhere private, you could do a move from yoga, Tai Chi or Pilates. Or you could wiggle your toes, tap your feet, shrug your shoulders, twiddle your thumbs, cup your hands, clench your buttocks, give yourself a gentle hug, slide your hands over your knees … and hundreds of other possibilities.

Once you've connected with your body, you move on to E — engage in what you're doing. You notice what you can see, hear, touch, taste or smell; notice where you are and what you're doing, and refocus on the task at hand.

I recommend you drop anchor:

- whenever an emotional storm blows up

- when you want to disrupt worrying, obsessing, ruminating — or any other thinking process that reels you in and pulls you out of your life

- when it's hard to focus on or engage in what you're doing; when you keep zoning out, drifting off or going onto autopilot

- when you're in fight-or-flight mode, gripped by anger or fear: dropping anchor is a great way to calm down — it doesn't magically get rid of those difficult feelings, but it does take the impact out of them; and it gives you control of your actions, so you can act calmly even though you don't feel it

- when you're in 'freeze' mode: shutting down, flopping, slumping, zoning out or disengaging (or in extreme cases, literally 'freezing up' — your body locking into position). Dropping anchor in 'freeze' mode will help to 'wake you up', energise you, give you back control of your actions, help you to engage in what you're doing.

Dropping anchor is an act of self-kindness: a caring and supportive way of responding to your suffering. So if you've been finding kind self-talk helpful, it's good to actively bring it into this exercise. For example, as you acknowledge your pain, you could say to yourself 'This really hurts. Hold yourself kindly.' (Or, better still, a catchphrase of your own.)

There are so many different options for dropping anchor, you can really tailor it to suit your own needs. As long as you're using the ACE formula, you're doing the exercise. You can do it as quickly or as slowly as you like, as often as you want, whatever you're feeling. And if you practise this regularly, it will pay big dividends in terms of health and wellbeing. It may take a while, though, so please persist and be patient; and remember these words, from the great Scottish author, Robert Louis Stevenson ...

66 Don't judge each day by the harvest you
reap, but by the seeds that you plant."

6

PSYCHOLOGICAL SMOG

Can you hear it? That voice inside your head? The one that virtually never shuts up? There's a popular misconception that folks who 'hear voices' are abnormal in some way, but we all have at least one voice inside our head, and most of us have quite a few! For example, most of us have at times been embroiled in an inner mental debate between the 'voice of reason and logic' and the 'voice of doom and gloom', or the 'voice of revenge' and the 'voice of forgiveness'. And we're all familiar with that self-judgmental voice that's often called the 'inner critic'. (I once asked a client, 'Have you heard of the "inner critic"?' 'Yes,' she said. 'I've got an inner committee!')

Obviously the ability to think is incredibly valuable, and it adds enormously to our quality of life. Without the ability to think, we could neither create nor appreciate books, movies, music or art; nor could we enjoy blissful daydreams, or plan for the future, or share our feelings with loved ones. However, a lot of our thoughts are not particularly useful. Suppose I plug into your mind, record all your thoughts for the next twenty-four hours and transcribe them onto paper. Then I ask you to read through the transcript and highlight any thoughts that had been *truly helpful* for you in responding effectively to the reality slap. What percentage of the thoughts on that paper do you think you would highlight?

For most of us, the percentage would be pretty small. It's almost as if the mind has a mind of its own; it seems to talk all day long about whatever it pleases, with little regard as to whether this helps us or not. In particular, it seems to be very fond of dwelling on pain from the past or worrying about the future or obsessing about problems in the present. And yet, even though what it has to say is often unhelpful, somehow it almost always manages to absorb us in its stories.

Before we go any further, let me clarify what I mean by 'stories' because sometimes people take offence at the word. All I mean by 'story' is a sequence of words or pictures that conveys information. I could use the more common term 'thoughts', or the technical term 'cognitions', but when we call them 'stories' this helps us to handle them more effectively. You see, our mind tells us all sorts of stories all day long. If they are 'true stories' we call them 'facts' — but facts make up only a tiny percentage of our thoughts. Our thoughts include all sorts of ideas, opinions, judgments, theories, goals, assumptions, daydreams, fantasies, predictions and beliefs that can hardly be called 'facts'. So the word 'story' doesn't imply that the thoughts are false or inaccurate or invalid. It's simply a way of describing what thoughts are: words or pictures that convey information.

I will be using the term 'story' frequently throughout this book, so if it's not a term you like then, please, every time you read it, replace it in your head with an alternative term such as 'cognition' or 'thought'.

Now consider this: how often does your mind keep you awake at night or consume huge chunks of your day with stories that induce guilt, fear, anger, anxiety, sadness, disappointment or despair? How often does it pull you into stories of blame, resentment, worry or regret? How often does it get you stressed out, wound up, angry or anxious, in a manner that makes your situation even harder?

If your answer to the last three questions is 'very often', then that shows you have a normal human mind. Yes, I did say 'normal'. That's what normal human minds naturally do. In Eastern philosophy they have known this for thousands of years but, somehow, in the West, we have bought into the idea that when the mind operates this way it is abnormal. This is very unfortunate because it sets us up to struggle with our minds (which is futile) or to judge ourselves harshly for the way we think (which is also futile).

Why our minds do what they do

It's a great irony that this wonderful instrument we call 'the human mind', which is so creative and innovative and immensely useful to us, came with an inbuilt tendency to judge, compare and criticise; to find fault, to focus on deficiencies, to see problems everywhere it looks.

If you're wondering why the human mind has this tendency, consider it in terms of our ancient ancestors. Many eons ago, the men and women who lived longest were those who could clearly see the current problems (e.g. dangerous animals, brutal weather and vicious rivals), those who could best anticipate future problems (e.g. *more* dangerous animals, brutal weather and vicious rivals), and those who could figure out how to solve these problems effectively. So if one of our ancient ancestors was wandering around in a perpetual state of bliss, thinking that everything was good enough as it was, seeing no problems and anticipating no problems, then he or she wouldn't have survived long enough to have children. Way before they reached puberty, they would have been wiped out by the dangerous animals, brutal weather or vicious rivals.

Thus, over countless generations our minds have become super-duper problem-solving machines. And everywhere the mind looks it sees problems: things that are *not good enough* the way they are. (So if anyone has ever told you that 'negative thinking' is a sign of a defective or weak mind, they don't know what they're talking about; it's a normal psychological process of a normal human mind.)

The great irony is, when our minds do unhelpful stuff like this they aren't trying to make life hard for us — they're actually trying very hard to help us: either to help us get something we want, or to protect us from something we don't want. Let's look at a few examples.

Worrying and predicting the worst. This is your mind trying to prepare you, to get you ready for action. It's saying, 'Look out. Bad things are likely to happen. You might get hurt. You might suffer. Get ready. Prepare yourself. Protect yourself.'

Ruminating and dwelling on the past. This is your mind trying to help you learn from past events. It's saying, 'Bad stuff happened. And if you don't learn from this, it might happen again. So figure out: why did it happen? What could you have done differently? Learn from this so you're ready and prepared and know what to do if something similar should ever happen again.'

Self-criticism, self-blame, self-judgment. Your mind is trying to protect you from failure or rejection or disappointment or broken relationships or health problems, or a bazillion-and-one other adverse outcomes. It gives you a hard time over things you've done or keep doing, because it wants you to stop; it predicts that if you keep on doing these things something bad is going to happen. Basically it's trying to help you do things better, so that you get better outcomes. Same deal when it judges you as a person: 'weak', 'defective', 'worthless', 'selfish', 'broken', 'unlovable' and so on. It's basically saying you need to change what you're doing — because if you carry on this way, bad stuff is going to happen: rejection, failure and so on.

Reason-giving. Your mind comes up with all sorts of reasons for why you can't change, shouldn't change or shouldn't even have to change. It may tell you that change is too hard, too painful, too scary; or you just don't have what it takes; or it's all hopeless — things can't possibly improve. Your mind is basically trying to protect you from getting hurt. It knows that if you step out of your comfort zone, take action to improve things, there's a risk you'll fail; and that will be painful. So again it's trying to save you from painful outcomes and adverse events.

Hopelessness, pointlessness, meaninglessness. Your mind says there's *no point trying* to improve things, because life itself is meaningless; just give up, stop caring about anything, treat life as pointless. Again, your mind is trying to save you from pain. If you can truly manage not to care about anything because it's all pointless/worthless/meaningless, that's going to save you from all the pain that comes when you *really do* care: all the pain of rejection and loss and failure, all that fear and anxiety that shows up when you step out of your comfort zone, all the frustration and disappointment when you don't get what you want. Basically, the message is 'Don't even try because you'll just get hurt even more.'

Suicidality. Here your mind is trying to save you from pain. Life seems unbearably painful, so your mind figures if you kill yourself, that will stop your suffering. (Note: suicidal thoughts are very common after intense reality slaps; however, this book isn't a treatment for suicidality. So if you are suicidal, please immediately seek professional advice.)

Blaming, revenge, resentment. Your mind is trying to save you from injustice and unfairness and bad treatment by others. So it points out what they've done wrong, or considers how to punish them. Its aim is to help you learn from these past events so you're better prepared to handle them in the future.

Self-doubt, insecurity. Many of us experience significant self-doubt or insecurity after a big reality slap. It may show up as doubt, indecision or lack of confidence in ourselves: 'Am I handling this the right way?', 'Am I making the right decisions, doing the right things? Or am I screwing it up?', 'Can I handle this?', 'Can I do this?' Again, this is your mind trying to protect you: watch out, be careful, this is new territory, there are new rules of play, you could get hurt. This may also manifest as questioning, 'Who am I?' This is very common after a major loss: 'Who am I without my job?', 'Who am I without a partner?', 'Who am I without my health?', 'Who am I without my parents?', 'Who am I without a child?' Here your mind is trying to help you think deeply about what sort of person you want to be, what values you want to live by, what you want to stand for in the face of your loss. (We'll be exploring these questions in depth in Part 2 of the book, 'Rebuild'.)

Vulnerability. We may also have a heightened sense of vulnerability. We just don't feel as strong or invincible as we used to. We might feel as if the world is not safe; that life is unpredictable; that bad things happen to good people; that we can no longer fully trust ourselves, or others, or the universe. These thoughts and feelings arise when our minds remind us of a truth we often forget: we *are* vulnerable, each and every one of us. Our minds are trying to tell us to look after ourselves, practise self-care, attend to our emotional, physical, psychological and spiritual health, and to do the same for our loved ones.

Foreboding, doom and death anxiety. When a reality slap involves death — or a close encounter with it — many people experience a sense of doom or foreboding, or an increased awareness of the inevitability of death for each and every one of us. This is your mind reminding you that life is precious and you never know how long you have left; so you need to make the most of it. (We'll look at how to do that in Part 3, 'Revitalise'.)

I'm going to stop there, but hopefully you get the point. Whatever unhelpful stuff your mind does, it's basically a misguided attempt to help you; to save you from pain, or help you get more of what you want. Have you ever had an 'overly helpful friend', one of those friends who's just trying so hard to help you they're actually becoming a nuisance? When your mind is churning out stories such as those listed above, see if you can think of it as 'an overly helpful friend' — it's trying hard to help you, but it's going about it the wrong way.

Cease the battle

Many popular psychology approaches encourage you to get into a battle with that voice in your head. They tell you to challenge, dispute or invalidate those 'negative' thoughts and replace them with 'positive' ones — and it's certainly a seductive proposition! It appeals to our commonsense: stomp on the 'bad' thoughts and replace them with 'good' ones. But the problem is, if we start a war with our own thoughts, we will never win. Why? Because there's an infinite number of those so-called 'negative' thoughts, and no human being has ever managed to find a way of eliminating them.

Zen masters, who are like the Olympic athletes of mind training, know this all too well. There's a classic Zen tale about an eager monk who asks his abbot, 'How can I find the greatest Zen master in the land?' The abbot replies, 'Find the man who claims he has eliminated all negative thoughts. And when you find this man ... you know that's not him!'

Yes, we can all learn to think more positively, but that won't stop our minds from generating all sorts of painful, unhelpful stories. Why not? Because learning to think more positively is like learning to speak a new language: if you learn to speak Hungarian, you won't suddenly forget how to speak English.

So if our only way of dealing with those thoughts is to battle with them — to challenge them in terms of whether they are true or false; to try to disprove them; to try to push them away, suppress them or distract ourselves from them; or to try to drown them out with more positive thoughts — then we will suffer unnecessarily. Why? Because all those popular 'commonsense' strategies require a huge amount of time and effort and energy, and for most people they really don't work too well in the long term. Usually what happens is the thoughts disappear for a while, but like zombies in a horror movie, they soon return.

A smoky haze

We have many ways of talking about this human tendency to get 'caught up' in our thoughts. We might use colourful metaphors like 'He's a million miles away', 'Her head's in the clouds' or 'He's lost in thought', or we might talk of worrying, ruminating, rehashing the past, stressing out, obsessing or being preoccupied.

Basically, this incredibly valuable, uniquely human ability to generate thoughts can leave us wandering around in a smoky haze, lost in our thoughts and missing out on life.

Of course, to be in a smoky haze is not necessarily bad. The smoky haze of incense sticks can be soothing and relaxing. The smoky haze of a bonfire can be exhilarating and fun. But what happens when the smoke gets too thick? You start to cough, your nose runs and your eyes water. And over time, if you keep on breathing in all that smoke you will eventually damage your lungs. Similarly, there's a time and place where being absorbed in our thoughts is life-enhancing: daydreaming on a beach, mentally rehearsing an important speech, creating new ideas for a project. But most of us get the balance wrong; we spend way too much time inside our minds, and we wander through our days in a thick cloud of 'psychological smog'.

And nothing thickens that smog like a big reality slap. The greater the discrepancy between the reality we've got and the reality we'd prefer to have, the more our minds protest. These protests may take a variety of forms. There might be denial ('This can't be happening') or anger ('This shouldn't have happened!') or despair ('I can't cope, I'll never get over this'). Our minds may agonise over the unfairness of it all; or compare our life to the lives of others and find it wanting; or conjure up all manner of terrible future scenarios. Our mind may go round and round in circles, trying to make sense of it all: 'Why me?', 'Why now?', 'How could this happen?', 'Why do bad things happen to good people?', 'What did I do to deserve this?' Our minds may tell us that 'Life sucks', 'This is unbearable', 'I'm too weak', 'I'm a bad person', 'I'm not getting over this fast enough', 'Life's too hard', 'It's my fault', 'They're to blame', 'You can't trust them' or thousands of other similar judgmental comments.

And as I've said before, these patterns of thinking are all very normal — they're just not very helpful. If we get caught up in these thoughts this will usually ramp up our struggle with reality and amplify the pain we're already feeling!

Now, before we go any further, I'd like to make one thing clear: *our thoughts are not the problem*. Our thoughts do not create 'psychological smog'. It is *the way we respond* to our thoughts that creates the smog. To understand what this means, let's consider …

What are thoughts?

In essence, thoughts are pictures and words in our heads. Don't take my word for this; check it out for yourself. Stop reading, and for 1 minute, close your eyes and notice your thoughts. Notice where they seem to be located, whether they are moving or still, and whether they are more like pictures, words or sounds. (Sometimes your mind goes shy when you attempt this; your thoughts disappear and refuse to come out. If this happens, just notice the empty space and the silence inside your head and wait patiently. Sooner or later your mind will start up again, even if only to say, 'I haven't got any thoughts!')

What did you notice? If your mind went blank at first, you would have noticed an empty space and silence, but eventually some thoughts showed up; and presumably those thoughts were words that you could see, sense or hear, or pictures you could see, or a combination of both. (If you noticed a sensation or feeling in your body, then that's exactly what it is: a 'sensation' or 'feeling'. Don't confuse those with 'thoughts'.)

When we allow these words and pictures to come and go freely, to flit through our awareness like birds in the sky, they create no problems. But when we hold onto them tightly *that* is when they turn into smog, *that* is when they pull us out of our life.

When we're lost in that smoky haze, all the details are obscured and all the richness is lost. We can't taste the sweetness for the smoke. On the other side of that smog, there might be the greatest show on earth — but we wouldn't know it. If you've ever spent some time inside this smog, you know how impenetrable it can be; even though we're surrounded by all sorts of opportunities to enhance and enrich our life, we are completely unable to see them.

Unhooking from our thoughts

There are many types of psychological smog and when we're in the thick of one we tend to fumble; it's hard to navigate our course and deal with the obstacles we encounter. In ACT we have a metaphorical name for this state; we refer to it as being 'hooked'. When our thoughts 'hook us' they dominate us; they reel us in, just like a fish on a line, and jerk us around, much like a puppet on a string. When we get hooked by our thoughts, they have an enormous impact on us; they seem to be commands we must obey, or threats we must avoid, or obstacles we need to eliminate, or something very important to which we must give our full attention.

In stark contrast, when we *unhook* from our thoughts they lose their power over us. *Unhooking* means we separate from our thoughts and see them for what they truly are: constructions of words and pictures. When we unhook from our thoughts they no longer dominate us; we don't have to obey them or give them all our attention; and we don't have to try to get rid of them. Instead, we see their true nature; we recognise that they are nothing more or less than words and pictures; and we allow them to come, stay and go in their own good time.

Naturally if our thoughts are *helpful* — if they help us to be kind and compassionate to ourselves, or to behave more like the sort of person we want to be, to make effective plans and take effective action to enrich and enhance our lives in practical ways — then we make good use of them. We don't let them *control* us — push us around, dictate what we do —but we do let them *guide* us.

When we adopt this approach to our thoughts, we are rarely if ever concerned as to whether or not they are true. What we're interested in is: are they helpful? If we give these thoughts all our attention or allow them to dictate what we do, will that *help* us adapt to our reality slap? If we let these thoughts guide us, will we act effectively, behaving like the sort of person we want to be? Or will it do the very opposite?

As Rada grappled with all the problems arising from her fibromyalgia, her mind would repeatedly trot out a litany of harsh self-critical thoughts: *Look how pathetic I am; I can't dance, can't cook, can't socialise, I'm useless.* Her previous therapist had tried hard to challenge these thoughts; to look for evidence to disprove them and replace them with more positive thoughts. This hadn't helped at all. I said to her, 'Your mind loves to give you a hard time, doesn't it?'

'I deserve it,' she said. 'Look how pathetic I am.'

'And when your mind beats you up that way, does it help you to deal with your condition?'

She paused for a moment, then answered softly, 'No.'

'Okay, so we are never going to get into a debate about whether your thoughts are true or false, or whether you deserve such harsh judgments. Instead, can we just acknowledge, a) those thoughts keep showing up, and b) when you get hooked by them, that makes life harder, not easier.'

'Okay.'

'Good. So, given that state of affairs, how about we work on some unhooking skills? Let's not debate whether these thoughts are true or not; let's just learn how to unhook from them.'

Of course, if our thoughts are helpful, we are wise to actively *use* them. (You'll see this clearly in Part 2 of the book, where we focus on taking action to rebuild our lives.) But if they're unhelpful it's best to unhook, to let them come and go, as if they are cars driving past our house.

If you're anywhere near a road right now, open your ears and see if you can hear the sounds of traffic. Sometimes there is a lot of traffic outside and sometimes there is very little. But what happens if we try to make the traffic stop? Can we do it? Can we magically wish it away? And what happens if we get angry at the traffic; if we pace up and down, ranting and raving about it? Does this help us live with the traffic? Isn't it easier just to let those cars come and go and invest our energy in something more useful?

And suppose a noisy old car drives slowly past your house, engine roaring, exhaust firing and loud music booming from within. You look out of the window and see the car is covered with rust and graffiti, and there's a group of young lads inside, singing along, whooping it up, shouting obscenities. What is the best thing to do? To run out of the house and start yelling at the car, 'Go away. You have no right to be here'? To patrol up and down the street all night long, to ensure the car doesn't come back? To attempt to keep such cars away in future, by asking the universe to provide only beautiful cars outside your house?

The easiest and simplest approach is to just let that car come and go: acknowledge it is present and allow it to pass on through in its own good time. To give you a sense of how to do this, here's ...

A simple three-step experiment

This experiment is quite similar to the book-pushing exercise in Chapter 4, but there are important differences, so please don't skip it.

Step 1: Imagine that in front of you right now is everything that's important in your life. This includes both the pleasant things — like the people you love, and all the movies, music, food, books, activities you enjoy — and the unpleasant things — like the challenges and problems you have to face up to and deal with. And imagine the book in your hands is made up of all the thoughts and memories that you find most difficult. (Take a few moments to name them.)

Step 2: When you reach the end of this paragraph, hold this book tightly around the edges, while keeping it open. Gripping the edges tightly, lift the open book up in front of your face, then bring it in so close that it's almost touching your nose — the book should be virtually wrapped around your face, completely obscuring your view of your surroundings. Hold it like that for about 20 seconds and notice what the experience is like.

What did you discover? While you were totally 'caught up' in your thoughts and memories, did you feel cut off and disconnected from the important things in your life? Did it seem as if your thoughts dominated everything?

This is what it is like when we are hooked by our thoughts and memories: we get lost in them, consumed by them or overwhelmed by them. They dominate our experience; make it hard for us to engage in or appreciate the enjoyable and pleasant aspects of life, or to respond effectively to the problems and challenges we face.

> **Step 3:** When you reach the end of this paragraph (again pretending this book is your thoughts and memories), place the book gently on your lap and let it sit there for 20 seconds. And as you let it sit there, stretch your arms, breathe deeply, and with a sense of genuine curiosity scan your surroundings and notice what you can see and hear around you.

Did you notice how it was much less distracting when the book was sitting on your lap; so much easier to focus on and engage in the world around you? Of course, it's easy to do this with a book; a whole lot harder with real thoughts. So, in the next chapter, let's do it for real!

7

NOTICE AND NAME

Have you ever walked around in *real* smog? When we're stumbling around in the *real* stuff, we know about it: it's hard to breathe, hard to see, hard to walk. But when we're lost in *psychological* smog we usually don't realise it, and sometimes we can be caught up in worrying, ruminating or obsessing for hours on end.

Thus, the first step in unhooking from our thoughts is simply *to notice* that we are hooked. This is a bit like suddenly glimpsing your reflection in a mirror and being surprised at your appearance; or catching and righting yourself just as you trip; or abruptly realising, in the middle of a conversation, that you haven't been listening to the other person and now you have no idea what they are talking about. It's an 'Aha!' moment; a gentle jolt; like suddenly waking up from a snooze.

I invite you to practise this often throughout the day. See if you can notice when and where your psychological smog arises: in your car, riding your bike, at work, at home, in bed, during dinner, playing with your kids, having a shower, talking to your partner, walking the dog? And try to recall what tends to precipitate the smog: an argument, a rejection, a failure, an unfair or dismissive act, a tight deadline, a great opportunity, a particular expression on somebody's face, a provocative comment, a piece of good news, a piece of bad news, a particular person, a song, a movie, a photograph, the mention of a loved one's name?

Also notice the kinds of smog that trap you. Common varieties include worrying, blaming, self-criticism, hopelessness, obsessing, wishful thinking, dwelling on problems, reliving horrors from the past, or predicting the worst for the future. This is useful information for the next step.

The art of naming

The second step in unhooking is to *name* the thought or thinking process in question; this generally gives us some distance from our thoughts. It's a bit like when you wake in fright from a nightmare. The first thing you do is notice that you're awake and in your bedroom. The next thing you do is name the experience: 'It was only a dream.' As you do this, you wake up further; the dream becomes more distant, the bedroom more present.

The good news is you've already learned how to do this, with the kind self-talk in Chapter 3 and the 'acknowledging' step when you drop anchor. The aim in this chapter is to develop this skill further, to ramp up its power and give it more 'oomph'. So, let's try this now with a thought that has a strong negative impact on you. Perhaps a harsh self-judgment like 'I'm bad', 'I'm worthless', 'I'm weak', 'I'm damaged goods'. Or perhaps a scary thought like 'I'm sick', 'I'll never recover', 'I can't keep going'.

Naming exercise

Once you've chosen your thought, you're ready to start the exercise.

Step 1: Say the thought to yourself, and let it hook you; buy into it as much as you possibly can.

Step 2: As soon as you have the sense that you are hooked, notice the thought and name it. Below are five different naming techniques, and I invite you to try all of them and see what works best:

- I'm having the thought that …

- I'm noticing the thought that …

- Here's my mind telling me that …

- I notice my mind telling me that …

- I notice I'm having the thought that …

Please try this now, before reading on. For example, if your mind keeps telling you that you're useless, then begin by taking a few seconds to let yourself get hooked. Say to yourself, 'I'm useless' and let it hook you; let it reel you in. Once you're hooked, say to yourself, 'I'm having the thought that "I'm useless"'. Try this with at least two or three different thoughts, and at least two or three different naming techniques, and notice what happens.

I hope you found that useful. When we notice and name a thought, we usually unhook from it, at least a little. However, that doesn't mean the thought disappears; sometimes it will, sometimes it won't. Nor does it mean we'll feel any better; sometimes we will, sometimes we won't. This isn't a technique to get rid of unwanted thoughts or control our feelings — so if we try using it that way, we'll soon be disappointed or frustrated. It's a way to take the power out of a thought, so it no longer dominates us, no longer pulls us into self-defeating behaviours or takes up all of our attention so we can't focus on or engage in what we are doing.

If this doesn't happen straight away, the next step is to drop anchor. We run through the ACE formula, and we bring naming into the 'acknowledge' component. As we acknowledge the thoughts that are present, we say, 'I'm noticing thoughts about being hopeless — and feelings of sadness and despair'. We then connect with our body and engage in what we're doing; and rinse and repeat as required.

Naming the pattern

Often there are so many thoughts whirring through our head it's not practical to name each and every one of them. In such cases, we're better to name the thinking pattern itself. For instance, when we notice we're all caught up in thoughts about things that might go wrong, we could name it 'worrying' or 'predicting the worst'. If we're dwelling on grievances and grudges, we might name that activity 'blaming' or 'resentment'. If we're going over our problems without reaching any useful outcomes, we might call it 'stewing' or 'ruminating'. If we're lost in painful memories, we might call it 'pulling me into the past'. If we're beating ourselves up, we might call it 'judging' or 'self-criticism'. And if you're not sure what to name it, you can always use the catch-all term 'thinking'.

Please play around with this concept. You may prefer phrases like: 'Here's my mind judging', 'Here's worrying', 'I'm noticing blaming', 'I'm noticing my mind pulling me into the past', 'Here's my mind hooking me', or perhaps simply 'Getting hooked'. The idea is to come up with a word or phrase that allows you to quickly name what your mind is doing. So here's how this might play out:

- First, you notice that you're hooked.

- Then you notice what's hooking you.

- And then you give that thought pattern a name: 'Aha! Here's worrying.'

- And as you name it, notice what it is: a construction of words and pictures.

- And then without trying to avoid or escape these thoughts, notice where you are and what you're doing.

And in that moment, you may notice a sense of lightness, as if the smog has thinned and you are now seeing the world with greater clarity.

And if that doesn't happen straight away, then run through your anchor-dropping routine:

A: acknowledge what's hooking you

C: connect with your body

E: engage in what you're doing.

This simple exercise is very empowering because it reminds us of where our true power lies: not in trying to stop these stories from arising; not in doing battle with them; but in stepping back, seeing them for what they are, and refocusing our attention where it's needed.

Naming the story

'Naming the story' is a popular alternative to naming the pattern. Imagine you are going to write a book or make a documentary about your current reality slap. And in some magical way you are going to put all your painful thoughts, feelings and memories into it. And you are going to give it a title that begins with the word 'the' and ends with the word 'story'. For example you might call it, the 'Life's Over' story or the 'Old and Lonely' story or the 'Never Get Over This' story. It needs to be a title that:

- summarises the main issue, and
- acknowledges that it is a huge source of pain in your life.

It can't be a title that mocks or trivialises the issue or makes fun of it. It can be a humorous title if you wish, but not a mocking or demeaning or trivialising one. (So if you try this technique and you end up feeling belittled or demeaned or invalidated, then please either change the title or forget this method and stick with naming the pattern.) Once you've come up with a title, use it to enhance the naming process: any time a thought, feeling or memory linked to this reality gap arises, notice it and name it. For instance, 'Aha! There it is again: the "Life's Over" story.'

A few years back, a middle-aged psychologist, let's call her Naomi, attended one of my workshops. During the mid-morning tea break Naomi confided in me that she had a malignant brain tumour. She had tried all the conventional medical treatments and many alternative ones as well (such as meditation, prayer, faith healing, creative visualisation, homeopathy, numerous diets and herbal remedies, positive thinking and self-hypnosis) but, sadly, the tumour was incurable and Naomi did not have much longer to live. She was attending my workshop to help herself cope with her fear, and to make the most of whatever life she had left. Naomi told me it was difficult to remain focused in the workshop. She was continually getting hooked by thoughts of death; she kept thinking of her loved ones and how they would react; she kept 'seeing' her MRI scans and that tumour spreading progressively through her brain; and she kept dwelling on the likely progression of her illness, from paralysis to coma, then death.

Now, clearly if we have a terminal illness, it's often helpful to think about the implications: to consider what we put in the will, and what sort of funeral we want, and what we wish to say to our loved ones, and what sort of medical care we need to arrange. But if you've gone to a workshop for personal growth, then it's unhelpful to be fused with such thoughts at that time; you will miss out on the workshop. So I listened compassionately to Naomi and, then, after first acknowledging how much pain she was in and empathising with her fear and validating how difficult it was for her, we talked about naming the story. (If I had leaped straight into this, chances are she would have felt upset or invalidated, as if I were trying to 'fix' or 'save' her without truly understanding or caring about just how much pain and difficulty she was in.) So Naomi came up with: the 'Scary Death' story.

I asked her to practise naming that story whenever she saw it coming, or whenever she became aware it had hooked her. She did this enthusiastically, and by lunchtime on day two of the workshop she was pretty unhooked from all those morbid thoughts. The thoughts had not altered in believability — she still considered them all to be true — but she was now able to let them come and go like passing cars and remain engaged in the workshop.

If you feel like it, you can even bring in some lightness and humour to this process. For instance, you might playfully say to yourself, 'Tut, tut, tut! It's just noooooooooot good enough!' or 'I guess The "Not Good Enough" show just started.' Or 'Aha! Here it is again. The old "I'm Weak" story. I know this one!' (But do be careful if you try this; if there's any sense of feeling belittled, mocked or trivialised, then drop the humour or go back to 'naming the pattern'.)

Thanking your mind

Earlier we discussed how the mind is like an 'overly helpful friend': trying hard to help but going about it in the wrong way. We explored how all that ruminating, worrying, self-judging, blaming, hopelessness and so on is basically your mind trying to save you from getting harmed or hurt. Knowing this, it can be helpful to 'thank your mind' for its input. For example, after you've noticed and named the thought, pattern or story, you might say to yourself — again, with a sense of playfulness — something like this: 'Thanks, mind. I know you're trying to help. And it's okay, I've got this covered. I'll deal with it myself.'

Not everyone finds this technique useful, but most people do. (It's one of my personal favourites.) Sometimes people say to me, 'Why should I thank my mind? It's making my life a misery!' I reply, 'It's just a playful way of taking the impact out of those thoughts. It's to help you take them less seriously, to stop fighting with them or trying to push them away.' But if they're not convinced, I don't try to persuade them; no technique is suitable for everyone. So I *do* encourage you to try this method and see how it works for you, because usually it helps us unhook a little bit more; but if it's not helpful, or you don't like the idea of it, give it a miss.

Neutralising

Noticing and naming our thoughts is usually enough to break their grip on us. If not, we can add anchor-dropping or thanking your mind, and that usually does the job. However, sometimes we need to go further and bring in something I like to call 'neutralising'. Basically, this involves doing something to our thoughts to 'neutralise' their power; something that helps us to see their true nature as a construction of words and pictures. Neutralisation techniques include silently singing your thoughts to popular tunes, saying them to yourself in different voices, drawing them in thought bubbles, visualising them on a computer screen, imagining them coming from cartoon characters or historical figures, and more. In Appendix A you'll find a number of these exercises, so if you feel like you need more help with unhooking from your thoughts, please go there and play around with the techniques before reading on.

We can't stop our minds from telling us stories, but we can learn to catch them in the act. And we can learn to choose the way we respond: to let the helpful stories guide us and the unhelpful ones come and go like passing cars.

8

LIVE AND LET BE

What's the big deal about breathing? Why do so many spiritual traditions get excited about it? In the Old Testament of the Bible, God formed man from the dust of the ground — and then breathed life into him through the nostrils. In ancient Greek mythology, the god Prometheus created man out of mud — and then the goddess Athene breathed life into him. As for the word 'spirit', this comes from the Latin *spiritus*, which means 'soul' or 'breath'. Likewise, in Hebrew the word *ruah* most commonly means 'breath' or 'wind', but also means 'soul'. Similarly, the Greek word *psyche*, from which we derive terms like 'psychology' and 'psychiatry', variously means 'soul', 'spirit' or 'breath'. And in the 'contemplative' or 'mystical' branches of all the world's most popular religions — including Christianity, Islam, Hinduism, Sikhism, Buddhism and Judaism — there are breathing exercises designed to help one access a higher state of awareness or a direct experience of the divine.

So how do we explain this strong connection between breath and spirituality? There are many contributing factors. First and foremost is the obvious link between breathing and life. As long as you're breathing, you're alive, which means there is always something purposeful you can do. Another factor is that breathing exercises are often quite soothing or relaxing. They can help us to access a sense of inner peace, to find a safe, calm place in the midst of an emotional storm. A third factor is that we can use our breath to anchor ourselves in the present. When we're all caught up in our thoughts and feelings, we can focus on our breath to ground ourselves and reconnect with our here-and-now experience.

We're about to explore two exercises that focus on breathing, but first, a few words of caution. Most people get a lot of benefit from these sorts of exercises, which is why you find them, in one form or another, in many self-help books. However, a small number of people have unpleasant reactions when they focus on or modify their breathing — such as dizziness, lightheadedness, pins and needles, a tight chest, or anxiety. These are very unlikely, but if any of these do happen, please do one of the following: a) if the exercise focuses mainly on the breath (such as the ones in this chapter), simply skip it; b) if breathing is *not* the main focus but there are a few instructions such as 'breathe into it' or 'take a slow breath' (as is the case with some exercises in later chapters), then simply ignore those instructions and do the rest of the exercise.

So now I'm going to invite you to do a brief exercise. You may be able to do this while still reading, or you may need to read the instructions first, then put the book down to do it.

Take a breath, hold and let go

Slowly take a large breath in and once your lungs are filled with air, hold your breath.

Hold the breath for as long as you possibly can.

Notice how, as you keep the breath trapped inside your body, the pressure steadily builds.

Notice what happens in your chest, neck and abdomen.

Notice the tension building and the pressure rising. Notice the changing feelings in your head, neck, shoulders, chest and abdomen. And hold that breath.

Keep holding.

Notice how the sensations grow stronger and more unpleasant; how your body tries ever more forcefully to make you exhale.

Observe those physical sensations as if you are a curious child who has never encountered anything like this before.

And when you can't hold your breath a moment longer, slowly and ever so gently release it.

And as you let it go, savour the experience. Appreciate the simple pleasure of breathing out. Notice the letting go.

Notice the release of tension.

Notice your lungs deflating and your shoulders dropping. Appreciate the simple pleasure of letting go.

How did you find that experience? Were you able to appreciate it? Did you notice a sense of grounding or centring yourself? Perhaps a sense of calmness or stillness?

How often in our day-to-day existence do we hold on to things, refusing stubbornly to let go? We hold on to old hurts, grudges and grievances. We hold on to unhelpful attitudes and prejudices. We hold on to notions of blame and unfairness. We hold on to self-limiting beliefs, old failures and painful memories. We hold on to unrealistic expectations of ourselves, the world or others. We hold on to stories of 'right' and 'wrong' and 'fair' and 'unfair', that pull us into fruitless struggles with reality.

Unfortunately, the phrase 'let it go' is often misunderstood. 'Let it go' doesn't mean 'make it go away' or 'get rid of those difficult thoughts and feelings'. It means loosen your grip on those thoughts and feelings, instead of holding on to them so tightly; and allow them to come and stay and go in their own good time, without getting caught up in them.

'Let it go' really means 'Let it be' — allow it to be as it is. In other words, instead of resisting, fighting, grappling with reality, we acknowledge this is how it is. We step out of the battle with reality because we know that reality always wins. This doesn't mean we give up on our lives; in Part 2 of this book the focus is on actively rebuilding our lives: taking effective action, doing whatever we can to improve them. It means we acknowledge that often when we're ruminating, worrying, obsessing, dwelling, entangled in our thoughts and feelings — that simply doesn't help. It doesn't alter what has happened; it doesn't change reality; it doesn't help us adapt to life as it is in this moment; and it doesn't help us to do anything effective in response to our problems and challenges.

Imagine if we could catch ourselves whenever we are holding on tightly to frustration, criticism, judgment, resentment or blame, and use our breath to remind us to 'ease off the grip'. What difference might that make to our relationships, our health and our vitality?

I now invite you to try another exercise, a little easier than the last one.

Take a breath, count to three

As slowly as you can, take a deep breath in. Then hold it for a count of three. And then, ever so slowly, gently exhale. Let the breath leave your lungs as slowly and gently as possible.

As you breathe out, let your shoulders drop and feel your shoulder blades sliding down your back.

And once again notice the sense of release.

Appreciate the simple pleasure of exhaling.

Notice what it's like to let ... it ... go.

Now do this one more time.

Slowly breathe in, then hold it for a count of three. And then, exhale as slowly and gently as possible.

And as you breathe out, let your shoulders drop.

And once again appreciate the simple pleasure of exhaling.

And notice what it's like to let ... it ... go.

I encourage you to try this exercise regularly throughout the day and see what difference it makes. Try it when you are holding on tightly to something — some hurt, resentment or blame that is draining away your vitality. Begin by noticing and naming what has hooked you: 'Here's blame' or 'I'm noticing anger' or 'Here's my mind dwelling on the past'. Then breathe, hold and exhale. Many people also find it helpful to silently say something like, 'Letting go' or 'Let it be'.

Suppose you're stewing over that fight you had with your partner, or replaying the unkind comments your boss made at work, or giving yourself a guilt trip about the way you lost your temper with the kids, dwelling on how unfairly life has treated you. These are all forms of 'holding on tightly'. And you don't need me to tell you that it doesn't help, that it merely increases your stress and drains your vitality. So once you notice yourself holding on, the next steps are really very simple: name what's hooking you, take a deep breath, hold it for three and then, very slowly ... let ... it ... go.

9

OUR ALLIES WITHIN

From out of the shadows, a deformed hand appears. Two of the fingers are missing their tips; the other two and the thumb are mere stumps. And between those two larger fingers there's a smoking cigar. And then the face of this smoker emerges from the darkness. It's a terrifying face covered with lumps, sores and swellings. And he asks, 'Do you like cigars?'

You may recognise this encounter, from an old movie called *Papillon*. It's a tense moment where the hero falls into a dark trench and finds himself face to face with a leper. As a child, this scene really frightened me. I had no idea what leprosy was, but I knew it was something dreadful and I was scared as hell I might catch it. It was only years later, at medical school, that I came to understand how leprosy causes such horrible disfigurations. Basically it's a bacterial infection, which has many adverse effects upon the body. And one of the worst effects is severe nerve damage to the arms and legs. The damaged nerves lose their ability to feel pain. And without this ability, you're in big trouble. Normally, when you place your hand on a sharp spike or a hot metal plate, the pain instantly makes you draw your hand away, thereby reducing your injury. Imagine how many injuries you'd sustain, and how much worse they would be, if you couldn't feel pain — if you left your hand resting on that spike or hotplate. With leprosy, these multiple injuries result in terrible damage to the hands, feet, fingers and toes, which brings us to the main point of this chapter: pain serves a purpose.

We've been talking a lot about pain in this book, which is understandable, given how much reality slaps hurt. So let's take a few moments to explore: *why do* we have all these painful thoughts and feelings? Are they just showing up to make us miserable? If not, what useful purpose do they serve?

In Chapter 6 we discussed this with regard to painful thoughts. We looked at how those painful things that minds do — such as worrying, ruminating and self-judging — all serve a purpose: our minds are trying to protect us, save us, look out for us. Similarly, in Chapter 1 we talked about how the nervous system clicks us into fight, flight or freeze mode to protect us from harm and danger. So we're now going to explore the three main purposes of our emotions ...

Communicate, motivate, illuminate

Our emotions are basically messengers that come to us with important information, trying to help us. They have three main purposes: communicate, motivate, illuminate.

Communicate

Let's start with communicate. When others can read our emotions, this is useful both for us and for them. (Assuming, of course, that they're not out to harm us or turn this information against us.) It allows us to communicate with each other in valuable ways. For example:

- Fear communicates 'Watch out; there's danger!' or 'I find you threatening'.

- Anger communicates 'This isn't fair or right' or 'You're trespassing on my territory' or 'I'm defending what's mine'.

- Sadness communicates 'I've lost something important'.

- Guilt communicates 'I've done something wrong and I want to put it right'.

- Love communicates 'I appreciate you'; 'I want you to stay close'.

When we're with people who care about us, people we can trust, these communications are often very valuable. For example, if a good friend sees you're scared or sad, she'll often respond with kindness and support. If she sees you feel guilty for something you did that hurt her, that'll often help to repair the damage done. If she sees you're angry about something she's doing, she might back off and reconsider it. Obviously there are times when we 'send the wrong signals' or others misinterpret them or react negatively; no system works perfectly. But most of the time, as a means of communication, emotions work pretty well.

Motivate

Our emotions also 'motivate'. The words 'emotion', 'motivate', 'motion' and 'move' all originate from the Latin word *movere*, which means 'to move'. Emotions prepare us to move our body in particular ways; to act in ways that are likely to be helpful and life-enhancing.

- Fear motivates us to run away, hide, take evasive action, protect ourselves.

- Anxiety motivates us to prepare ourselves for things that might hurt or harm us.

- Anger motivates us to stand our ground, to fight for what we care about.

- Sadness motivates us to slow down, ease up, take a break from the demands of everyday life, rest up and recuperate.

- Guilt motivates us to reflect on our behaviour and how it's affecting others, and to make amends if we've hurt them.

- Love motivates us to be loving and nurturing, to share and to care.

Again, this is an imperfect system. At times these emotions show up when they aren't helpful and they hook us, and pull us into problematic behaviours. But a lot of the time these emotions do work pretty well, provided we don't struggle with them. If we start fighting with or running from these emotions, we create big problems for ourselves. Remember the book-pushing exercise in Chapter 4? Pushing it away with all your strength ate up your energy, distracted you, made it hard to act effectively. And that's what happens when we fight with or run from our emotions. But if we drop the struggle with them, make room for them, let them flow through us — as you'll learn to do in the next chapter — we'll find we can often make use of them in life-enhancing ways.

Illuminate

Last but not least, our emotions illuminate what's important to us. They alert us that there is something going on that matters, something we need to attend to. They 'shine a light' on our deepest needs and wants. For example:

- Fear illuminates the importance of safety and protection.
- Anger illuminates the importance of defending our territory, protecting a boundary or standing up and fighting for what is ours.
- Sadness illuminates the importance of rest and recuperation after a loss.
- Guilt illuminates the importance of how we treat others and the need to repair social bonds.
- Love illuminates the importance of connection, intimacy, bonding, caring and sharing.

In other words, there's a whole lot of wisdom in our emotions. We can't access this wisdom when we're fighting with them or distracting ourselves from them, but once we learn how to open up and make room for them (in the next chapter) then it's a different story. And later we'll look at how to extract this wisdom — from both our thoughts and feelings — and actually use it to help us rebuild our lives.

Hopefully you're starting to see that our emotions are our allies, not our enemies. And the more we turn away from them, the more we miss out.

Missing out

66 Mr Duffy lived a short distance from his body."
– James Joyce, *Dubliners*

I love this quote. To be honest, I haven't read *Dubliners*, so I've no idea why Mr Duffy lived a short distance from his body, but I can tell you he's not the only one. Most of us are at times very disconnected from our bodies — especially when they're full of painful feelings. This makes sense. We'd stay out of the water if we knew there was a great white shark in there. Similarly, we like to 'stay out' of our bodies if we know we'll encounter painful feelings in there.

At times, the autonomic nervous system makes this decision for us: 'cuts off' our emotions, leaving numbness in their place. But, more commonly, we choose to numb ourselves: with medication, drugs or alcohol. And, most commonly of all, we escape from our bodies through distraction. The word 'distraction' comes from two Latin words: *dis*, which means 'apart', and *trahere* which means 'to draw'. So when we talk about 'distracting ourselves', we mean that we 'draw apart' from something unpleasant or unwanted. When we distract ourselves from painful feelings, we 'draw apart' from the body that houses them.

The more we lose touch with our bodies — whether through substance use, distraction or involuntary numbing by the vagus nerve — the more problems this causes. Perhaps the most common is the awful sense of lifelessness it fosters. People variously describe this with words and phrases such as numb, empty, hollow, dead inside, an empty husk, a shell, a zombie, a walking corpse, feeling nothing, half alive, barely alive, or lifeless. These words describe a state that is the very opposite of 'vitality'.

The word vitality comes from the Latin *vita*, meaning 'life'. Vitality refers to the life force within us: our energy, drive and passion; our appreciation of life; our ability to feel fully alive and participate fully in the world. Our bodies keep us alive, and our feelings remind us we're alive; so it's hardly surprising that when we disconnect from them we lose that sense of vitality.

But the problems don't stop there. A wealth of scientific research shows that when we cut off from our bodies we lose that emotional wisdom we discussed above, which in turn leads us to suffer in many ways. For example:

- We have less control over our impulses and urges, which makes us more prone to behaviours such as aggression, drug and alcohol abuse, or overeating.
- We lack self-awareness and our judgment is impaired, often leading to 'bad decisions', which we later regret.
- We have difficulty reading the emotions of others, which, combined with lack of self-awareness, gives rise to conflict and tension in relationships.
- We have difficulty being intimate with others, which leads to disconnection and loneliness.

Many people are surprised about these side effects of emotional disconnection, so I'd like to briefly explain why they happen.

Kids in the classroom and pictures on TV

Remember when you were a kid and your teacher left the classroom? What happened? All hell broke loose, right? Well, it's the same thing with our emotions. Our awareness is like the teacher, and our emotions are like the kids. If we're not aware of our feelings they play up, create havoc, run riot. The less aware we are of our feelings, the more they control our actions; they jerk us around like a puppet on a string and easily pull us in to problematic patterns of behaviour. When the teacher returns to the classroom, the kids immediately settle down. Same deal when we bring awareness to our feelings; they lose their impact and their ability to jerk us around.

Of course, when the teacher's out of the classroom, she's got no idea what the kids are up to. And it's much the same for us when we disconnect from our feelings; we call this 'lacking self-awareness'. Did someone close to you ever say something like this: 'You seem in a bad mood', 'Why are you so grumpy?', 'You seem down', 'Are you okay?' If so, did it take you by surprise? Did you say, 'I'm not' or 'No, I'm fine!' Did you ever catch yourself raising your voice or being snappy without knowing why? Or overeating, or drinking too much, or crying a lot — all for 'no obvious reason'? Or making decisions that you later judged as 'stupid' and wondered 'Why did I do that?' These common scenarios all point to a lack of emotional awareness.

As we go about our day, interacting with others, our body continuously generates feelings based on what is happening; and these feelings are a goldmine of information provided we are able to access them. So, to switch metaphors for a moment, have you ever watched a movie without the sound on? (If you haven't, please try it for a minute.) How diminished is the experience? The images are great — but without the music, the dialogue, the sound effects, we lose so much. We can still track what's happening to some extent, but without any sound it's a much less satisfying experience and we can easily misread or lose track of what's going on. And this is just what it's like when we interact with others while cut off from our own emotions. Our relationships suffer because we misread other people; we misread their intentions, misread their feelings; fail to pick up on what they want or don't want, or lose track of how our own words and actions are affecting them.

Finally, consider love and intimacy. Loving, intimate connections within a loving, caring relationship usually give rise to pleasurable feelings; but if we're cut off from our body we won't get to enjoy them.

Instead, in those situations we'll feel numb or empty. This makes intimate connection an unpleasant experience — which then feeds into *dis*connection and loneliness — and often leads to avoidance of intimacy.

So the more you 'stay away' from your body, the less access you have to your emotions, which places you at a huge disadvantage — so the problems caused by your reality slap only accumulate. It's hardly surprising that a wealth of scientific research shows that 'getting back into our bodies' makes a huge difference to our health and wellbeing (and plays a central role in recovery from trauma). This is why in dropping anchor, you repeatedly 'acknowledge your feelings' and 'connect with your body'. Moving, stretching, breathing, altering your posture — these are all simple, practical ways to connect with your body throughout the day. (But these brief actions are only the start; as you'll see later in the book, we can go much further.)

Mind and body

In summary then, when your mind and body generate all these painful thoughts and feelings, they're actually trying to help you. All that discomfort they generate — all those difficult thoughts, all those fight-and-flight responses, all those painful emotions and feelings, and all that numbness and emptiness — all stems from one overarching purpose: your mind and body are working hard to protect you, to save you from getting hurt or harmed.

'That's all very well,' you may be thinking. 'But I still don't like it.' And I agree with you. No one likes pain and discomfort. No one wants it, no one chooses it. Reality slapped you around and your mind and body responded the best way they know how. You didn't ask for all this suffering; life dumped it on you. And it really hurts. And when life hurts this badly, kindness is called for. To run away from our feelings is not a kind way to treat ourselves, because it creates so many problems in the long term. What we need is a radically different way of responding to difficult feelings — which is the focus of our next chapter.

In the meantime, I hope this chapter has encouraged you to start looking at your emotions in a different way. Please do keep on noticing and naming them — 'Here's sadness', 'I'm noticing anger', 'I'm having feelings of guilt', etc. *And* at the same time, even if you don't yet fully understand what it is, see if you can also acknowledge that they serve a purpose. You might even silently say to yourself 'These emotions aren't out to get me; they're here to help.'

10

A CURIOUS LOOK

A wave of nausea washes over you. Your eyesight becomes blurry and foggy, and within a few seconds, it completely disappears. Your throat is paralysed almost instantly, preventing you from speaking or swallowing. And over the next two to three minutes this paralysis spreads throughout your body until you can no longer breathe. This is how your life would end if you were bitten by the tiny bird-like beak of the deadly blue-ringed octopus, an organism no bigger than a tennis ball.

A good friend of mine, Paddy Spruce, likes to ask the question, 'If you were swimming near a blue-ringed octopus, would you pick it up, chase it away, ignore it or simply observe it?' Clearly, all these options are available to us, but the first two are deadly, and while this octopus is not naturally aggressive, if you try to pick it up or threaten it in any way, it will bite. (Just before it attacks, you will see the blue rings on its tentacles suddenly light up.) As for the third option — ignoring it — that would be pretty hard to do, knowing how deadly it is. Plus, if you don't pay attention to where it is, you might accidentally swim into it.

So, the last option, observing it, is clearly the best. 'Hang on a minute,' you might be thinking. 'There's another option you didn't mention. I could swim away from it.' Yes, you could. However, the blue-ringed octopus prefers to hide under rocks rather than swim in the open, so if you stay still and observe, it will soon pass on by and leave you alone. And even if you choose to swim away, wouldn't you first want to get a good look at it, knowing that as long as you don't try to pick it up or threaten it, you are perfectly safe?

This tiny sea creature provides a good analogy for a painful emotion: if you hold on to it, chase it away or try to ignore it, the results are usually bad. Unfortunately, many of us treat our emotions as if they are as dangerous as that octopus. We want to get rid of them or avoid them. We can't be at ease when they're around. We try to figure out how to make them go away. And this attitude, unfortunately, absorbs a lot of our energy and drains our vitality.

However, it doesn't have to be that way. Why? Because unlike the octopus our feelings are *not* dangerous. If we stay still and observe our emotions with curiosity, then they cannot hurt us or harm us in any way; and like that blue-ringed octopus, sooner or later they will pass.

Now, suppose you were a marine biologist and you had paid a small fortune for the opportunity to observe the blue-ringed octopus in its natural environment. Under those circumstances, knowing you were safe, you'd observe that creature with absolute fascination. You'd be curious about its every move. You'd notice the rhythmic movements of its tentacles; you'd notice the beautiful patterns and colours on its body; and you'd respect it as a magnificent work of nature. And it's this type of open, curious attention that helps take the impact out of our emotions. In other words, when a painful feeling arises we don't have to get sucked into it and we don't need to fight it or run from it. Instead, we can observe it, make room for it, and allow it to come, stay and go in its own good time. And if your mind has something unhelpful to say about that prospect — a protest, threat, worry, judgment or some other form of resistance — then please let it have its say and carry on reading.

Feelings, emotions and sensations

As many people get confused about the differences between feelings, emotions and sensations, it's worth taking a moment to clarify them. The hardest term to clarify is 'feelings' because it's used in so many ways. It's commonly used as another word for emotions, such as feelings of sadness or anger (I often use it this way in the book). But it's also used for physiological states — feelings of thirst, hunger, sickness or tiredness. Most commonly of all, it's used as a synonym for 'sensations' — meaning anything that we feel in our physical body, whether that's the tightness in our chest when we're anxious or that burning in our fingers when we accidentally touch a hot stove, or those feelings of numbness when freeze mode kicks in.

The term 'emotions' is also hard to clarify because most experts can't completely agree on what they are. But there are some things they do agree on. For example, almost everyone agrees that emotions communicate, motivate and illuminate. Also, on a physical level, an emotion includes neurological changes (i.e. involving the brain and nervous system), cardiovascular changes (i.e. involving the heart and circulatory system) and hormonal changes (i.e. involving the 'chemical messengers' of the blood). However, while we can measure these changes on scientific instruments, this is not how we experience our own emotions. When we look at our emotions with open, curious attention, all we will ever encounter are thoughts and sensations. (Remember: 'thoughts' are words and pictures inside our head; 'sensations' are what we feel inside our body.)

The best way to make sense of this is to check it out for yourself: observe your emotions with curiosity. As you do this, you will either notice something comprised of sensations or something comprised of words and pictures. Or rather, you will notice complex, interweaving, multilayered tapestries of pictures, words and sensations. And you can zoom in on specific thoughts or sensations, or you can zoom out and take in the whole spectacle.

To make this clearer, consider your favourite movie. If you were to watch a 1-second segment of that film, all you would encounter are sounds and pictures. We wouldn't call any one of those sounds or pictures a movie in itself; and we wouldn't say a movie is nothing but 'sounds and pictures'. But, *experientially*, when you look at any second of any movie, all you will encounter are sounds and pictures. You can think of an emotion similarly: a rich, compelling, multilayered creation comprised of many, many interweaving sensations and thoughts.

When we pay attention to the threatening, unpleasant or painful stuff inside us — to all those thoughts and feelings that we normally turn away from — and when we are willing to take a good honest look at it all and really examine it with openness and curiosity, then we are likely to discover something useful. We learn that it is not as big as it seems; that we can make room for it. We learn that it cannot harm us, even though it feels unpleasant. We learn that it cannot control our arms and legs, even though it may make us shiver and shake. We learn that there is no need to run and hide from it, nor to fight and struggle with it. This frees us up to invest time and energy in improving our life rather than in trying to control the way we feel. Without genuine curiosity, it is unlikely we will ever discover this.

Normally, when painful feelings arise we are not curious about them. We have no desire to get up close and study them and see what they are comprised of. We have no particular interest in learning from them. Generally speaking, we don't want to know about them at all. We want to forget about them, distract ourselves from them or get rid of them as fast as possible. Rather than take a close look at them, we instinctively turn away. It is much the same as the way we automatically recoil or avert our gaze from the sight of a diseased or deformed body. And yet, as automatic as it is, this is a response that we can change with practice.

Working as a doctor, I have had the opportunity to see many different ways in which the human body can become deformed: through blistering skin diseases, the terrible scarring of burns, the merciless rampages of cancer and AIDS, the distorted swollen joints of immune disorders, the missing limbs that result from surgical amputations, the misshapen heads and twisted spines of rare genetic disorders, the bloated abdomens and yellowing flesh of liver disease, and the myriad forms of physical deterioration associated with old age, illness and death.

Before I entered the medical profession I felt a sense of shock, fear, aversion or disgust whenever I saw people with these conditions. But over the years, I gradually learned to see past the unpleasant exterior and connect with the human being inside. I learned to pay attention with warmth, curiosity and openness and, over time, my aversion and fear disappeared and in its place came kindness and compassion. However, this only happened through my willingness to be present and open up; to make room for my automatic emotional reactions without letting them control me. If we are willing, we are all capable of making this transition.

At this point, let's note that there are two very different types of curiosity. There is a cold, detached, uncaring curiosity, such as that of a lab scientist doing experiments on a rat or monkey. And then there is a warm, caring curiosity, such as that of a kindly vet trying to work out how to heal a sick animal. You've probably met some doctors who are cold and detached, curious only about the illness, interested only in the diagnosis and treatment. They seem to care very little about the human being inside that afflicted body. And you've probably met other doctors who are the opposite: warm, kind and caring in their curiosity. They care first and foremost about the human being; they treat the whole person, not just the condition. Which kind of doctor would you prefer to have treating you?

The word 'curiosity' originates from the Latin term *curiosus*, which means 'careful' or 'diligent'. This, in turn, comes from the Latin word *cura*, which means 'care'. I find this very interesting. When practising self-compassion, we are caring for ourselves; we care about what we feel and we care about how we respond to our feelings. Avoidance of our feelings is, in contrast, often an uncaring act. We get so focused on trying any way possible to get rid of them that we end up harming ourselves or shrinking our lives in the process. The word *cura* also gives us the word 'cure' and this seems appropriate because curiosity plays such an essential role in emotional healing; instead of trying to escape from our pain we turn towards it, investigate it, explore it and, ultimately, make room for it. This is a true act of caring and healing.

So, next time loneliness, resentment, anxiety, guilt, sadness, anger or fear shows up, what if you could become really curious about those experiences? What if you could shine a light on them, study them as if they were the prize exhibit in a show?

As we look more curiously into any intense stress or discomfort, we will find that it is comprised of two major components. One is the storyline: all those words and pictures inside our heads — beliefs, ideas, assumptions, reasons, rules, judgments, impressions, interpretations, images and memories. The other is our body sense: all those feelings and sensations inside our body — which is what we're going to focus on next.

Making room

Yes, you guessed it — time for another exercise. We're going to learn how to open up and make room for difficult feelings such as anger, sadness, guilt, fear, loneliness, numbness and emptiness. But, first, pause — and notice what your mind has to say. Is it enthusiastic, curious, eager? Or is it protesting: 'No! I want to get rid of these feelings, not make room for them!'

If the latter, your mind has probably forgotten why we're about to do this important work. Remember Chapter 4, where we looked at all the things you've done to avoid these feelings, and how that works short-term but not long-term? How the more effort and energy you expend in trying to avoid and get rid of these feelings, the more tired and drained you are, the harder it is to act effectively in the face of all your hardships, and the harder it is to engage in any aspect of life? And remember last chapter, where we looked at the costs of cutting off from our emotions? Learning how to drop the struggle with your feelings and let them freely flow through you is an act of self-kindness. You're not doing this work 'just for the sake of it'; you're doing it so you can start rebuilding your life.

Before we start the exercise, a few practicalities. First, two quick reminders. One: if you'd like my voice as a guide, download the free audio from *Extra Bits*. Number two: if you have any difficulties with breathing exercises, such as those we discussed in Chapter 8, then ignore any instruction to do with your breath.

Second, you'll note the exercise begins with anchor-dropping. That's essential; please don't skip it. And if at any point the exercise becomes overwhelming (I'm not expecting this; just being cautious) then please stop doing it, and drop anchor until you are once again grounded.

Third, it's okay to do this in baby steps. No one expects a firefighter to tackle a towering inferno without any training. The trainee firefighter practises on small, safe fires, lit under carefully controlled conditions within specially designed training grounds. Only when she's done lots and lots of practice, knows her equipment inside out, knows all the drills and manoeuvres — only then will she go out and fight real fires.

A similar approach is wise when it comes to making room for difficult feelings. So, if you've never tried anything like this before, don't begin with your most overwhelming emotions. Start with those smaller, less challenging feelings: the hundred different forms of impatience, frustration, disappointment, sadness and anxiety that arise as part of everyday living. If necessary, you can start with just one small sensation, somewhere in your body. And then, gradually, over time, work up to bigger ones.

Notice your feeling

Take a few moments to drop anchor. Do this in your own manner, acknowledging your inner experience, connecting with your body, engaging in the world around you, until you have a sense that you're grounded.

Then pause for a moment.

You are about to embark on a voyage of discovery; to explore a difficult feeling and see it with new eyes. If no such feeling is present, then see if you can bring one up: take a few moments to reflect on the nature of your reality slap and the way it is currently affecting you. Usually as you do this, difficult feelings will arise.

Take a slow, gentle breath and focus your attention on your body.

Start at the top of your head and scan downwards. Notice where in your body this feeling is strongest: your forehead, eyes, jaw, mouth, throat, neck, shoulders, chest, abdomen, pelvis, buttocks, arms or legs? (If you're numb, focus on wherever the numbness is most evident: often the chest or abdomen.)

Once you have located a difficult feeling, observe it with wide-eyed curiosity, as if you are a marine biologist who has encountered some fascinating new denizen of the deep. See if you can discover something new about it — about where it is, what it feels like, or how it behaves.

Notice its energy, pulsation or vibration. Notice the different 'layers' within it.

Notice where it starts and stops.

Is it deep within you or at the surface? Moving or still?

Imagine this feeling as an object inside you: what is its shape and size? Is it light or heavy?

What is its temperature? Can you notice hot spots or cold spots within it?

What is its colour? Is it transparent or opaque?

If you could touch the surface of this object, what would it feel like?

Hot or cold? Soft or hard? Rough or smooth?

Notice any resistance you may have to it. Is your body tensing up around it? Is your mind protesting or fretting?

Name your feeling

As you notice your feeling, name it. Silently say to yourself, 'Here's fear' or 'I'm noticing anger' or 'I'm having a feeling of guilt'. (If you can't pinpoint the exact name of the feeling, then try 'Here's pain' or 'Here's stress' or 'Here's numbness'.)

And continue to observe this feeling, as if it is some fascinating sea creature. The big difference now is this creature has a name; you know what you are dealing with.

Breathe into your feeling

Breathe slowly and deeply, and imagine your breath flowing into and around the emotion.

And as your breath does this, it's as if in some way you expand — as if a space opens up inside you.

This is the space of awareness.

And just as the ocean has room for all its inhabitants, your own spacious awareness can easily contain all your emotions.

So breathe into the feeling and open around it. Loosen up around it. Give it space.

Breathe into any resistance within your body: the tension, the knots, the contraction; and make space for all of that too.

Breathe into any resistance from your mind: the smoky haze of 'No' or 'Bad' or 'Go away'.

And as you release the breath, also release your thoughts. Instead of holding onto them, let them come and go like leaves in the breeze.

Allow your feeling

There is no need to like, want or approve of this feeling. Just see if you can allow it.

Remember: this feeling serves a purpose; this is your body trying to help you.

This feeling tells you something very important.

It tells you that you care; that you have a heart; that there's something that really matters to you.

It's not a sign of weakness, or mental illness. It's a sign that you're a normal, living, caring human being.

And it's something you have in common with every living, caring human being; we all experience reality slaps, and we all have painful feelings when they happen.

So can you drop the struggle and make peace with it?

This feeling is a part of you. It's just as much a part of you as your hands and feet, your eyes and ears.

What do you get for going into battle with parts of yourself? Can you step out of that battle and make peace?

And as you continue to observe this feeling, see if there's anything underneath it. For example, if anger or numbness is at the surface, perhaps underneath it is fear, sadness or shame. But don't try to make a new feeling appear; just allow your feelings to be as they are in this moment. If a new feeling 'emerges from the deep', that's okay; and if it doesn't, that too is okay.

Whatever feeling is there in this moment, let it have its space. Give it plenty of room to move. And allow it to come and go freely, in its own good time.

Expand your awareness

The marine biologist may concentrate her attention on the octopus, but she can also broaden her focus to notice the water around it and the rocks beneath it.

And we can all widen our focus in a similar way. Thus, once you've made space for your feeling, the aim is to expand your awareness. Continue to notice your feeling and, at the same time, recognise it is only one aspect of the here and now.

Around this feeling is your body, and with that body you can see, hear, touch, taste and smell.

So, take a step back and admire the view; do not only notice what you are feeling but also what you are hearing, seeing and touching.

Think of your awareness as the beam of a powerful torch, revealing what lies hidden in the darkness. Shine it in all directions, to get a clear sense of where you are.

As you do this, do not try to distract yourself from this feeling.

And do not try to ignore it. Keep it in your awareness, while at the same time, connecting with the world around you.

Allow the feeling to be there, along with everything else that is also present.

Notice what you are feeling and thinking.

Notice what you are doing and how you are breathing. Notice it all. Take it all in.

Straddle two worlds with your awareness: the one within you and the one outside you. Illuminate both with your consciousness.

And engage fully in life as it is in this moment.

As with all exercises in this book, you can practise this any time, any place, for any duration. For example, if you want to improve your ability to make room for difficult emotions, you could stretch this into a long exercise, taking a good 10 to 15 minutes. On the other hand, you can practise a 10- to 15-second version just about anywhere: simply notice and name the emotion, breathe into it, allow it to be there, and expand your awareness to connect with the world around you. You can also mix 'making room' with other exercises. For example, after noticing, naming and allowing your feeling, it's great to finish up with some kind self-talk or dropping anchor.

Now perhaps you may be wondering, '*What's next? After I finish this practice, what do I do?*' The answer is, if you're doing something purposeful and life-enhancing, keep doing it and engage in it fully; focus all your attention on the task at hand and become thoroughly absorbed in it. And if you're *not* doing something purposeful and life-enhancing, then stop what you're doing and switch to an activity that's more meaningful. (And if you can't think of any meaningful activities, don't worry, we'll get to that in Part 2.)

At this point, an important reminder. Emotion control strategies — all those things you do to escape, avoid or get rid of unwanted feelings — are only problematic if and when you use them excessively, when they're giving you relief in the short term but impairing your life in the long term. So if they're helping you cope and not adversely affecting your life in the long run, then it makes sense to keep using them. What we're trying to do here is enlarge your toolkit, to give you more options so you don't have to go through life always fighting with or running from your feelings, or cutting off from your body to escape them.

I encourage you to make the effort, at least several times a day, to take a good curious look at your feelings. Watch your feelings closely and discover their habits. When do they appear? What brings them out? Which parts of your body do they like to occupy? And how does your body react to them? Where do you notice the resistance, the tension and the struggle?

When watching a documentary, we can be thrilled at the sight of a shark or a crocodile or a stingray. These deadly, vicious creatures can fill us with awe and appreciation. Our challenge is to view our emotions in much the same way. For, although our feelings might appear to be dangerous, they are actually unable to harm us in any way. Unlike a shark or a crocodile, they cannot eat us. Unlike a stingray, they cannot poison us. When we watch our feelings with openness and curiosity, that's no more dangerous than watching a wildlife documentary. So take a curious look, whenever you can. It doesn't have to be a long look, just a curious one.

11

A KIND HAND

You've got a pet donkey, right? And every weekend, your donkey carries your goods to the marketplace for you to sell there. No? Oh. Oh well, never mind. Even if you don't have a donkey of your own, I'm sure you know that donkeys are renowned for being stubborn. So if you want your donkey to be cooperative, you need to know how to motivate it. And if you're wondering what on earth this has to do with reality slaps, you'll find out very shortly.

Often reality slaps are forced upon us, through death, disease and disaster. At other times we create those slaps ourselves, at least in part, through our own self-defeating behaviour. We all screw up, get it wrong and make foolish mistakes. We all, at times, get jerked around by our emotions like a puppet on a string, and act in self-defeating ways. Entangled in our thoughts and struggling with our feelings, we end up saying and doing things that are far removed from the person we really want to be. We might hurt the people we love the most, or we might avoid them because we feel we are unworthy of their love.

As we practise and apply the principles within this book, we'll find this sort of thing happens less often, but the fact is we will never be perfect. We will screw up again and again and again. This is part of being human.

So what does your mind tend to do when you screw up? If it's anything like my mind, it pulls out a big stick and starts whacking you; it tells you you're *not good enough*, or you can't do it, or there's something wrong with you; or it lectures you about the need to try harder, to do better and improve yourself. And this is hardly surprising. When we were growing up, adults often criticised us in an attempt to get us to change our behaviour; no wonder then that we grow up doing this to ourselves.

Now, let's return to that donkey I mentioned earlier. You've probably heard the old saying about 'carrot versus stick'. If you want to get a donkey to carry your load, you can motivate it with a carrot or a stick. Both approaches will get the donkey moving but, over time, the more you hit that donkey with the stick, the more miserable and unhealthy it becomes. On the other hand, if you reward the donkey with a carrot whenever it does what you want, then over time you end up with a much healthier donkey (with really good night vision). Beating yourself up, coming down hard on yourself or getting stuck into yourself is just as ineffective as hitting a donkey with the stick. Sure, harsh self-criticism will sometimes get you moving in the right direction, but the more habitual it becomes, the more miserable and unhealthy you will be. It's highly unlikely to help you change your behaviour; it's far more likely to keep you feeling stuck and miserable.

So whether our reality slap came about by sheer bad luck, or whether we in some way contributed to it, practising self-compassion is essential. (Unless, of course, you want to go through life like a battered donkey; somehow I doubt that.)

By the way, the skills you've been learning in the last few chapters — dropping anchor, unhooking from unhelpful stories, making room for difficult emotions — are all technically known as 'mindfulness skills'. And given that 'mindfulness' is such a big part of the ACT model, you may be wondering why I haven't mentioned the term until now. The reason is simply because there are so many false notions about mindfulness; people think it's a religious practice, or a type of meditation, or a relaxation technique, or a form of positive thinking. Hopefully by now you can see that none of those ideas are correct. 'Mindfulness' is a term with many different definitions, and there's no universal agreement as to which definition is best.

Personally, I define 'mindfulness' as: 'A set of psychological skills for effective living — which all involve paying attention with openness, curiosity and flexibility'. When we are dropping anchor, unhooking from unhelpful stories, making room for difficult emotions, we are responding *flexibly* to our experience, *paying attention* to what is present with an attitude of *openness* and *curiosity*; in other words, we are practising mindfulness.

Of course, some people are far more mindful than others: far more able to focus on and engage in what they are doing, to open up and make room for their feelings, and to unhook from their thoughts. And this is largely due to the amount of practice they do. So far in this book I've only spoken about informal practice: quick and simple mindfulness exercises you can readily do throughout the day, virtually any time, any place. However, if you'd like to really develop your capacity for mindfulness, you may also want to consider a formal practice, such as 'mindfulness meditation' or Hatha yoga or Tai Chi.

There's one particular formal practice that is very useful and I highly recommend it: mindfulness of the breath. It involves focusing attention on your breathing and bringing your attention back repeatedly, no matter how often it wanders. In Appendix B you'll find a detailed description of the exercise. A word of warning, though: if you've never done an exercise like this before, you will be shocked at how challenging it is. If you can stay focused on your breath for even 10 seconds before your attention wanders to something else, you'll be doing well.

All the mindfulness skills we've covered so far are important elements of self-compassion; they are all kind ways of responding to your reality slap, kind ways of handling painful thoughts, feelings and memories. And what we're going to do next is blend these mindfulness skills together, along with some kind words and kind actions, to give you the full experience of self-compassion. (And yes, there's an audio in *Extra Bits*.) Some of my clients — especially men — are initially reluctant to do this next exercise; they protest that it's 'silly', 'flowery' or 'touchy-feely'. But once they get past those judgments and give it a go, they usually find it helpful (Antonio certainly did, as you'll see).

A kind hand

Find a comfortable position in which you are centred and alert. For example, if you're seated in a chair you could lean slightly forwards, straighten your back, drop your shoulders and press your feet gently onto the floor.

Take a few moments to drop anchor. Do this in your own manner, acknowledging your inner experience, connecting with your body, engaging in the world around you, until you have a sense that you're grounded.

Now bring to mind your reality slap. Take a few moments to reflect on what has happened, and notice what thoughts and feelings arise.

Be present.

Pause.

That's all you need do: just pause.

Pause for a few seconds and notice what your mind is telling you. Notice its choice of words, and the speed and volume of its speech.

Be curious: is this story old and familiar, or is it something new? What time zones is your mind taking you into: the past, present or future? What judgments is it making? What labels is it using?

Don't try to debate with your mind or try to silence it; you'll only stir it up.

Simply notice the story it's telling you.

And notice, with curiosity, all the different feelings that arise in your body. What do you discover? Guilt, sadness, anger, fear or embarrassment? Resentment, despair, anguish, rage or anxiety? Numbness, emptiness, apathy? Pay attention, like a curious child, to what is going on inside in your body.

And name these feelings as they arise: 'Here's fear', 'Here's sadness', 'Here's numbness'.

And say something compassionate to yourself: acknowledge your pain and respond with kindness. If you're not sure what to say, try 'This is difficult. Hold yourself kindly.'

Open up

Now find the feeling that bothers you the most and observe it like a curious child.

Where is it located? Is it at the surface or deep inside?

What is the size and shape of it? Are its borders well defined or vague and fuzzy?

What's the temperature of this feeling? Can you notice any hot spots or cold spots within it?

Is it moving or still? Light, heavy or weightless?

Can you notice any other sensations within it? Vibrating, tingling or throbbing? Pressure, burning or cutting?

Now slowly and gently breathe into the feeling, with an attitude of warmth and kindness.

Imagine your breath flowing into it and around this pain or numbness.

Imagine that in some magical way, a vast space opens up inside you, making plenty of room for this difficult feeling.

No matter how unwanted this feeling may be, do not fight with it. Step out of the battle. Instead, make peace with it.

Let this feeling be as it is. Give it plenty of space, rather than pushing it away.

And if you notice any resistance in your body — tightening, contraction or tension — breathe into that too. Make room for it.

Make space for all that arises: your thoughts, your feelings and your resistance.

Hold yourself kindly

Now choose one of your hands.

Imagine this is the hand of someone very kind and caring.

Place this hand, slowly and gently, either on your heart or on the feeling. And if you don't wish to touch your body, then instead let your hand hover above the area where the feeling is.

Perhaps you feel this more in your chest, or perhaps in your head, neck or stomach? Wherever it is bothers you most, lay your hand there. (And if you can't locate any particular place, then rest or hover your hand over your heart.)

Let your hand rest there, lightly and gently.

And sense its warmth flowing into your body.

Imagine your body softening around the pain, loosening up and making space.

Hold this pain or numbness gently. Hold it as if it is a crying baby or a whimpering puppy, or a fragile work of art.

Infuse this gentle action with caring and warmth, as if reaching out to support someone you care about.

Let the kindness flow from your fingers.

Now, use both of your hands. Place one of them upon your chest and the other upon your stomach, and let them gently rest there. Hold yourself kindly and gently: connecting with yourself, caring for yourself, giving comfort and support.

Speak kindly

Now again, say a few kind words yourself.

If you're not sure what to say, try 'This is difficult; hold yourself kindly.'

Or you might say, 'This is difficult — and I can do this.'

If you've failed or made a mistake, then you might like to remind yourself, 'Yes, I'm human. Like everybody else on the planet, I fail and I make mistakes.'

And acknowledge that your pain tells you something very important.

It tells you that you have a heart; that you care; and you've lost something or someone that really matters to you.

And this is what all humans feel in the face of great loss.

It's not a sign of weakness or of something wrong with you; it's a sign that you're a living, caring being. And it's something you have in common with every living, caring being on the planet.

As Antonio did this exercise with me, a guttural growl of anguish broke from his throat. His body heaved, and tears poured down his face. I asked him gently to keep his hands on his body, continue sending in kindness. And he did. He stayed that way for a good 10 minutes, sobbing, shaking and holding himself kindly. Eventually, his crying stopped and a calmness came over him. He looked at me sheepishly, said in a hushed voice, 'I've been trying so fucking hard not to feel that.'

'And now, how do you feel?'

'Like I just had ten kinds of shit kicked out of me!'

'You seem a lot calmer,' I said. The angst and tension he'd brought into the session had evaporated; he looked peaceful.

'Yeah — I guess I am,' he said, and smiled.

Antonio's reaction to the kind hand exercise was dramatic. For most people, that doesn't happen. More commonly, you'll tap into a sense of warmth and comfort. It's soothing and calming, and tends to centre and quiet you. If you do tap into some strong painful emotions, there's a choice to make. One option is to end the exercise and drop anchor. The other option is to keep going with the exercise and 'ride the storm'. Then, when the storm eventually subsides, you'll probably be in a similar state to Antonio; you'll feel like you've been through a lot — perhaps a bit shaky or vulnerable — but you'll also have a sense of calmness or comfort.

So I encourage you to do this exercise repeatedly — at least once a day (but even once a week is beneficial). And if it feels too long, you can easily strip it down into a 2-minute version.

Obviously this wouldn't go down well in the middle of a business meeting; it is best to keep this as something you do in private! It's also great to do in bed, especially if you can't sleep. And if by some chance you didn't get much out of it, please try it at least one more time. With repetition, most people find it helpful. (However, if you don't want to do this exercise, or you don't get anything out of it, or if it triggers a negative reaction that's too overwhelming for you to handle — just leave it.)

Also feel free to adapt or modify this exercise. For example, if you don't like placing your hands as suggested above, you can substitute another gesture of kindness such as rubbing your neck or shoulders, or massaging your temples or eyelids. And if you're doing a regular grieving practice, it's often very helpful to include this exercise as a part of it.

Going further

Aside from practising this exercise, what other acts of kindness can you do for yourself? How about making time for your favourite pastime, whether that's playing sport or tinkering with your car or reading books or working out in the gym? Or having a soothing warm bath? Getting a massage? Eating some delicious healthy food? Going for a walk? Giving yourself some 'me time'? Listening to your favourite music?

Can you listen to yourself non-judgmentally and acknowledge the extent of your suffering? Can you treat yourself gently and give yourself the benefit of the doubt? Can you recognise you're a fallible human being so of course you make mistakes? Can you look for the goodness in yourself? (It is definitely in there, no matter how much your mind may deny it.)

We've touched a few times on kind self-talk, and I want to explore this a bit further. As you know, there's no delete button in the brain; we can't magically eliminate all those harsh self-judgmental thoughts. But we can acknowledge and notice and name them when they show up, and allow them to be there without letting them jerk us around. And we can also generate kind, helpful thoughts to support ourselves. But the way we do this in ACT is very different to most other psychological approaches. We don't try to challenge, dispute, disprove or get rid of those self-critical thoughts; we don't try to turn 'negative thoughts' into 'positive' ones. Instead we acknowledge the judgmental thoughts, allow them to be present — *and in addition* we bring in some kind self-talk; we speak to ourselves the same way we would to a good friend in need.

For example, suppose your mind says, 'I'm so weak. Why can't I be stronger? Why I can't handle this as well as other people?' You might then respond like this: 'I'm noticing thoughts about being weak. And the fact is, this really hurts, and I'm struggling — but even though it's difficult, I can handle this. I'll take it one day at a time, and I'll focus on what's in my control.'

Or suppose your mind says you are a bad mother/father/son/daughter/friend because you weren't there for a loved one in their time of need, or you weren't able to save them from something bad, or you treated them badly in some way — and it gets stuck into you with all sorts of nasty self-judgments. You might respond with: 'Here's the "I Screwed Up" story. And the truth is, there are lots of things I regret, and I wish I could go back in time and do things differently — and it really hurts like hell that I can't. But beating myself up won't change what happened. What I can do, though, is learn from this, so I can act differently if something similar ever happens again.'

Notice how with these responses there's no self-pity going on; nor is there any attempt to deny or dismiss your very real pain. And there's no trite positive thinking going on: 'If life gives you lemons, make lemonade', 'Look at the glass half full', etc. They're all elaborations on that basic two-step formula: acknowledge your pain, respond with kindness.

Of course, this is a lot easier said than done: as we'd expect, like any new skill, self-compassion takes practice. But also, like any new skill, it does get easier with practice. So see if throughout the day you can find opportunities to run through the drill: notice and name your harsh, self-judgmental thoughts and allow them to be present. Then consider: if you wanted to be kind and supportive to a loved one who was going through something similar to yourself, what would you say?

Think small

To develop self-compassion, we don't have to do something big and dramatic. The tiniest act of kindness makes a difference. For example, here are a few acts I have done this morning: I stretched my back and neck, I had a hot shower, I played with the dog, I joked around with my son, I ate a healthy breakfast, and I listened to the birds outside the window. Such tiny acts of caring build up over time into a supportive, compassionate relationship with yourself. And even if you just *imagine* doing these acts, then that in itself can generate a sense of self-kindness.

Earlier in the book I mentioned Kristin Neff, the world's top researcher on self-compassion. Neff identifies three core elements of self-compassion: mindfulness, kindness and 'common humanity'. Neff's phrase 'common humanity' refers to the human condition and the universal nature of suffering. When we are hurting and suffering, let's remind ourselves that these are *normal* human experiences; that all over the planet, in this moment, there are millions upon millions of other human beings suffering in ways very similar to our own. We don't do this to discount or trivialise our pain, but rather to acknowledge it as part of being human; as something we have in common with everyone else; as something that can help us to understand the suffering of others and extend our compassion to them too.

Often when we're suffering, our mind tells us that we are the only one. That everybody else out there is happier than we are! That others don't feel the pain that we feel. That others don't experience major losses — at least, not to the same extent as ours. And if we buy this story, it will make our suffering all the more intense. The reality is, all humans suffer. Every human life will be touched by loss and hardship. Everybody gets reality slaps — many, many times if they live long enough. And it's often useful to remind ourselves of this, as part of our kind self-talk.

Personally, I find self-compassion hardest on those occasions when I have yelled at my son. Like all parents, at times I lose my temper. Hooked by some judgmental story, I lose touch with my values of patience and calmness, and I snap and say harsh words. Moments later, my mind comes out with the big stick: 'Bad father!', 'What a lousy job you're doing!', 'He's just a kid, go easy on him; what are you losing your temper for?', 'Call yourself an ACT therapist? What a hypocrite you are!', 'What would the readers of your books think if they could see you now?' And before I know it, I am flailing around in an emotional storm of guilt, embarrassment and frustration.

And then ... after a while ... I realise what is going on and I plant my feet onto the floor and I take some deep breaths and I notice what I can see, hear, touch, taste and smell. I connect with the world; I get present. And I acknowledge that I am hurting. And then I gently place a hand on my chest or my abdomen — wherever it hurts the most — and I breathe deeply. And I remind myself: 'You're a human being. And like every other parent on the planet, you screw up sometimes. This is what it feels like when you really care about being a good parent and you don't manage to live up to your own ideals.'

And then I look deeper at what's underneath all that guilt. And there it is: LOVE. Sheer, boundless love. After all, if I didn't love him I wouldn't have any guilt about yelling at him.

And if you make the time to sit quietly, to be kind and gentle with yourself and take a curious look at your emotional pain, then I suspect you will find something similar inside yourself. Whatever the emotion is — anger, fear, sadness or guilt — hold it gently and ask yourself 'What does this pain reveal about my heart? What does it remind me that I really care about? What does it tell me that I need to face up to, or deal with, or do differently?'

These questions help you to remember that you are not 'bad', even if your mind says you are. You are a caring human being. After all, if you didn't care, you wouldn't hurt.

So, when reality knocks us around, and turns our life upside down, dropping anchor and holding ourselves kindly are usually the best places to start. They help us to regroup after the blow; to get back on our feet and collect ourselves. After that, we'll be far more effective when we move into strategising and problem-solving: taking action, guided by our values, to start the painful process of rebuilding. So throughout your day, as well as repeatedly dropping anchor, look for opportunities to practise tiny acts of self-kindness. Each and every one of them makes a difference.

12

WHEN MEMORIES HURT

Sometimes the sweetest, richest memories can give rise to the most painful emotions. This is especially so when we've lost someone we love through death, separation or relationship breakdown. Because as we remember the good times — all those moments of love and play, intimacy and connection, sharing and caring — the enormity of our loss confronts us. And all of a sudden, that sweet joyful memory is awash with sadness, or anxiety, or loneliness — or a hundred and one other painful feelings. And that's the good memories! When the bad ones show up, we suffer all the more. Because there's no love or sweetness in the bad ones; there's only more pain.

In this chapter, we'll look at two different yet somewhat connected strategies. First, we'll explore 'acknowledging loss' practices for working with the pain of good memories; then we'll explore 'giving support' exercises for coping with the pain of the bad ones.

Groundwork

The good news is, you've already done some solid groundwork for what comes next. You've been dropping anchor when painful memories show up; an excellent first step for any painful inner experience. And you've also been noticing and naming them: 'I'm noticing a memory of the funeral', 'I'm having a memory of the car accident', 'I notice my mind remembering how she held me', 'Here's a memory of my boss giving me the sack'.

You've also been using kind self-talk: acknowledging how painful the memory is and responding with kindness; as well as 'making room' for the painful feelings that show up. You've been 'unhooking' from all those self-judgmental stories: 'I'm having the thought that I screwed up', 'Here's my mind telling me that I'm weak', 'I'm noticing the "Damaged Goods" story'.

Hopefully you've found these practices have already made a big difference; that you're able to acknowledge those memories and allow them to be present while you engage in what you're doing. And hopefully you've also noticed that like every other element of an emotional storm, your memories come and stay and go in their own good time. (And if you haven't been practising these things — well, now is a great time to start.) So, building on those skills, let's now take a look at …

'Acknowledging loss' practices

When someone you love dies, 'acknowledging loss' practices are usually of great value. (We'll talk shortly about how to modify these exercises for other types of loss, such as your job, your health or your relationship — but first we'll focus on bereavement.) The idea is to create a routine or ceremony that you do on a regular basis, which helps you over time to come to terms with your loss. There are no hard or fast rules about how to do this, how long to do it for, or how often to do it; it's really up to you to experiment. Many people find it helpful to include most or all of the following elements.

A regular time and place

Many people find there's something very comforting in doing this practice regularly: same time, same place. You might visit a graveyard or go to a beach or forest, or visit a place of worship, or use a room in your house. You might do this daily, weekly or monthly. You might take 5 minutes, an hour, or half a day. There are no rules; experiment and find what works for you.

A strong reminder

It's often helpful to have something present that strongly reminds you of your loved one: a photograph or painting, an item of their clothing, a toy or teddy bear they loved.

A symbolic act

The idea here is to do something that symbolises your love for this person. For example, this may involve lighting a candle, laying flowers on a grave, playing a special piece of music, reading a poem, saying a prayer, or writing in a journal. And if another person is participating, you might hold their hand, or hug them, or sing or pray together.

Remembering and allowing

During this time, the aim is to remember your loved one and allow your feelings to be as they are. Make room for all the thoughts and feelings that arise: love and sadness; joy and fear; laughter and loneliness. And acknowledge how much it hurts, and treat yourself kindly. Many people find it soothing to practise the kind hands exercise from the previous chapter as they do this.

Keep in mind that unwanted memories may appear. If this happens, it's important that you don't try to push them away, because doing so usually results in a rebound effect; the unwanted memories disappear for a short while, then bounce back with a vengeance. So if an unwanted memory shows up, notice it, name it, allow it — and hold yourself kindly.

Choosing memories

We have very little control over our memories. They tend to come and go as they please. Often they appear when we don't want them; at other times we can't retrieve them, no matter how we try. However, during a grieving ritual, you can choose to focus on certain memories that you want to hold dear. It's worth taking some time to consider how you want to remember this person. For example, were there particular occasions or events that were really special? Things they said or did that really mattered to you? Quirks of their personality you found endearing? Or personal qualities you admired? If so, you might like to consciously relive and reflect on these beautiful moments, and savour the sweetness within them.

Talking with your loved one

Last but not least, many people find it useful to talk to their loved one. If you've never done this, it might sound odd; after all, your loved one is dead. Yet these imaginary conversations are often very healing. If you want to experiment with this, you may choose to speak aloud or in your head. You may like to talk to your loved one about old times, or tell them things you wish you'd said before they died, or keep them informed of what is now happening in your life. And if you wish, you can also imagine them talking back to you.

Natalie, whose son died in the hit-and-run, was quite religious. She had a twice-weekly practice of visiting her son's grave — and during those visits, she prayed, and spoke to him, and laid flowers upon his tombstone. In addition, every night she would light a candle in his bedroom and pick up an item of his clothing. She would practise the kind hands exercise — holding the clothing against her body, underneath her hands — and let herself cry. Then she'd finish up with a prayer.

Antonio and Cathy created a grieving practice where once a week they'd go into baby Sophia's bedroom, stand in front of her crib, and hold hands. They'd light a candle, play some music and take it in turns to share with each other their fondest memories of their beautiful baby girl. Usually they'd end up sobbing and hugging each other tightly.

It's hard to overestimate the power of these 'acknowledging loss' practices (also known as 'grieving rituals'). They are not for everyone (so it's fine if you prefer to skip them) but most people find them very comforting — even though they are often very painful. Given that you never quite know what's going to show up as you do them, it's a good idea to kick off with dropping anchor; and bring it in again as often as you need to. And of course, like everything else in this book, the idea is to experiment and find what works for you.

For other types of loss — losing your job, or your health, or an important relationship — these practices can also be useful, but usually they're a lot more low key. For example, Shanti's practice, following the bust-up of her marriage, was to sit on the couch for 10 minutes every night, acknowledge her heartbreak, make room for all the memories that surfaced, and practise the kind hands exercise. Rada's practice — acknowledging all that she had lost as a result of her chronic illness — was almost identical to Shanti's, except she preferred to do it in the morning before getting out of bed.

'Giving support' exercises

How do we deal with really awful memories? Memories loaded with threat, danger, violence, death, disaster? Well, first things first: all those skills we discussed earlier in the chapter (under the heading 'Groundwork') are very important. And if you've been practising them, you've probably already found these awful memories are having less impact. 'Giving support' exercises offer a way to reduce that impact even further. These are essentially exercises in imagination. You imagine yourself travelling back in time to soon after the bad event happened, and then you imagine giving yourself the support you didn't have at that time.

For example, the first time he did this, Antonio imagined himself travelling back in time to the day after the death of baby Sophia. In his imagination, the Antonio of now stood beside the Antonio back then, placed an arm around his shoulders, and spoke to him in a kind and comforting manner.

Emily had been in a horrific car accident that crushed her pelvis and scarred her legs. So she imagined that the Emily of now travelled back in time to give support to the Emily back then (four months prior), arriving at the moment she was finally removed from the mangled car. The Emily of now comforted the Emily back then, held her hand in the ambulance and stayed by her bedside in hospital.

Note that in these exercises, *you don't go back to the actual awful event*. The reason for this is that it's often too overwhelming to do this alone. If you're having flashbacks or extremely distressing memories, the wisest move is to work with a well-trained therapist who is skilled in a process called exposure; this involves working directly with the memories, with lots of guidance and support from the therapist.

So instead of going back to the actual event, you go back to sometime *after* it occurred. And, once there, you give yourself support in any way you want. Most people use compassionate words and gestures, but it's your imagination so you can do whatever you like — as long as it's kind and supportive.

I'm going to take you through one of these giving exercises now, but please — *don't* work with your current reality slap. You're not yet ready for it. The aim at this point is to learn what's involved by working with a memory from a long time ago. After that, you can try this with something more recent. (And if you want my voice to guide you, you know the drill: download the audio from *Extra Bits*.)

As usual, this exercise begins with dropping anchor. And if at any point something overwhelming happens (not expecting it — just being cautious) please stop the exercise and drop anchor.

Giving support to the 'younger you'

You are about to do an exercise in imagination. Some people imagine with vivid, colourful pictures, much like those on a TV screen; others imagine with vague, fuzzy, unclear pictures; while others imagine without using pictures at all, relying more on words and ideas. However you imagine is just fine.

You're going to imagine travelling back in time to visit a younger version of yourself, at some point in your life when you were struggling, and the people around you were for one reason or another unable to give you the care and support you needed. This could be when you were a child, or more recently as a teenager or young adult.

Find a comfortable position and spend a few moments dropping anchor: acknowledging what's going on in your inner world, connecting with your body through moving or stretching or breathing, and engaging in the world around you: noticing what you can see, hear and touch.

Once you're grounded, either close your eyes or fix on a spot, and allow yourself to imagine.

Imagine yourself getting into a time machine. And once inside that machine, you travel back in time to visit your younger self. Find the 'younger you' at some point in their life when they are struggling and the adults around them, for one reason or another, are not providing the care and support they need.

Now step out of the time machine and make contact with the younger you. Take a good look at this child, teenager or young adult and get a sense of what s/he is going through. Is she crying? Is he angry or frightened? Does she feel guilty or ashamed? What does this young person really need: love, kindness, understanding, forgiveness, acceptance?

In a kind, calm and gentle voice, tell this younger you that you know what has happened, that you know what he's been through; that you know how much she is hurting.

Tell this younger you that he doesn't need anyone else to validate that experience because *you* know.

Tell this younger you that she got through this difficult patch in her life and it is now a distant memory.

Tell this younger you that you are here, that you know how much this truly hurts and you want to help in any way you can.

Ask this young person if there's anything she needs or wants from you — and whatever she asks for, give it to her. If he asks you to take him somewhere special, go ahead and do it. Offer a hug, a kiss, words of kindness or a gift of some sort. This is an exercise in imagination, so you can give her anything she wants. If this younger you doesn't know what he wants or doesn't trust you, then let him know that's fine; he doesn't need to say or do anything.

Tell this young person anything you think he needs to hear, to help him understand what has happened — and, if he's been blaming himself, to help him stop doing so.

Tell her that you are here for her, that you care, and you'll do whatever you can to help her get through this.

Continue to radiate caring and kindness towards this younger you in any way you can think of: through words, gestures, deeds — or if you prefer, through magic or telepathy.

Once you have a sense that this younger you has accepted your caring and kindness, it's time to bid farewell. Give him a gift of some sort to symbolise the connection between you. This might be a toy or teddy bear for a younger child; for someone older, perhaps an item of clothing, a book, a magical object, or anything else that springs to mind.

Say goodbye and let her know that you'll come back to visit her again. Then get in your time machine and come back to the present.

And now drop anchor for a minute or so. Acknowledge what's showing up inside you. Connect with your body — have a good long stretch. And engage with the world around you: use your eyes and ears, and notice where you are and what you're doing.

I hope you found that exercise helpful. And now you know what's involved, you can adapt it to your most recent reality slap. Like Antonio and Emily, you can go back and visit yourself in the hours, days, weeks, months (or even years) that followed the event. And, just as for a grieving practice, it's useful to do this regularly; indeed, on each occasion you do it, you might choose to visit a different point in time.

Please play around with both these practices, which you can see are both infused with self-compassion. Tweak the exercises in any way you like; adapt and modify them to suit your unique situation. And, of course, if they aren't helpful for you then skip them. Instead, keep noticing, naming, and dropping anchor whenever painful memories arise. There's no 'delete button' in the brain; no way to eliminate painful memories. But, over time, as you treat yourself kindly and allow your memories to be present without a struggle, you're likely to notice two things: they'll appear less often, and they'll steadily lose their impact.

This brings us to the end of Part 1 of this book. Before moving on to Part 2, you might want to take a few weeks to really work on the skills we've covered so far:

- dropping anchor amidst emotional storms
- opening up and making room for difficult feelings
- unhooking from harsh self-talk
- acknowledging your pain and responding with kindness.

To regroup after a reality slap is usually not a quick and simple process. The bigger the slap, the harder you fall and the deeper the wounds you sustain. And deep wounds don't heal quickly. Emotional storms will continue to arise. Your mind will continue to tell you unhelpful stories. And there will be many times when you forget everything we've covered so far in this book. But ... you can get better at remembering. And in that moment when you remember, you have a choice. You can, if you wish, drop anchor, acknowledge your pain, and respond to yourself with kindness. And each and every time you make that choice ... a little healing happens.

PART 2
REBUILD

13

MAKING LIFE MEANINGFUL

Without any sense of meaning, life lacks colour and richness. It's like living in black and white. There's little or no joy or satisfaction. And the odd thing about reality slaps is that they can either fill our lives with meaning — reminding us what truly matters, connecting us deeply with our heart — or they can drain it all away, leaving us empty and dissatisfied. All too often it's the latter rather than the former, at least during the immediate aftermath. So our aim in this next section of the book is to see if we can turn that around. And if your mind says that's impossible, that's a perfectly natural reaction. Because the truth is it takes time, effort and courage to start rebuilding your life after a reality slap, as well as a whole lot of patience.

The problem is, the harder reality slaps us the less motivated we are to even think about rebuilding. We're often so exhausted and drained that even the thought of taking action brings up anxiety or dread. So it's important to go slow and think small; take baby steps. Have you ever built a brick wall? No, me neither. But I'm sure you've seen bricklayers in action, and you'll have noticed that when building a wall you can't simultaneously lay twenty different bricks. You lay one brick at a time. First one. Then another. And then another. And so on.

The same principle applies to rebuilding your life. You don't try to work on every aspect of your life simultaneously; that's a recipe for getting overwhelmed and hopeless. The idea is to focus on one small aspect of life at a time. Let's start this off by exploring a very important question …

What's the point?

Every action we take serves a purpose. From doing the washing to eating an ice-cream; from getting married to filling in a tax return; from zoning out in front of late-night TV to going for an early morning jog. Underlying each and every action, there is always some sort of intention — we are taking action to make something happen. But how often are we conscious of this intention? And how often do our actions *consciously* serve some greater purpose that personally matters to us?

For most of us the answer to both questions is: 'not too often'. Our tendency is to go through life on autopilot, rather than consciously choosing what we do and how we go about doing it. The problem with this is that we could end up spending large chunks of our days acting in ways that are largely unfulfilling. However, if we consciously align our actions to a cause that is personally important then everything changes. Our life becomes imbued with meaning. We develop a sense of direction, of behaving like the person we want to be. And we experience a sense of vitality that is wholly missing from life on autopilot.

In the ACT model, this process of making life meaningful is called 'living by your values'. Values are basically your heart's deepest desires for how you want to behave as a human being. They describe what sort of person you want to be; how you want to treat yourself and others; and how you want to treat the world around you. They are like an inner compass that can guide you as you go on life's long and winding journey. And they are also like an energy source: they can motivate and inspire you to do the things that matter, even when you don't feel like it.

What follows is a quick exercise to help you start thinking about your values. But before you start, it's important to know there are no such things as 'right values' or 'wrong values'. It's like your taste in ice-cream. If your favourite flavour is chocolate but someone else prefers vanilla, that doesn't mean that their taste in ice-cream is right and yours is wrong, or vice-versa. It simply means you have different tastes. Similarly, we all have different values.

Values

This exercise involves simply reading a list of forty common values — not the 'right' or 'best' ones, just ones that many people share. The idea is to read through the list and see if any of these resonate with you. (Perhaps all of them will resonate; perhaps none of them. It's not a test; just an exercise to get you thinking about values.) Please read the list slowly, and pause for 2 seconds after each word to consider whether this word describes how you would like to behave towards yourself, others or the world around you, if you could choose to do so.

I'd like to behave in ways that are:

Accepting	Adventurous	Assertive
Authentic	Attentive	Caring
Committed	Compassionate	Cooperative

Courageous	Creative	Curious
Engaged	Fair	Focused
Friendly	Forgiving	Fun-loving
Generous	Genuine	Grateful
Helpful	Honest	Humorous
Kind	Loving	Mindful
Open	Playful	Reliable
Respectful	Responsible	Self-caring
Self-protective	Self-supportive	Sincere
Supportive	Trusting	Trustworthy
Understanding		

If some of those words describe how you'd like to treat yourself or others or the world around you, then in the ACT model we'd call them your 'values'. (But if there are words there that do *not* describe how you want to behave, then they are not your values — and that's okay.)

Upon the vast table of our life we find many different dishes; some are exquisitely pleasurable, others are intensely painful. When reality slaps us around, pleasurable dishes are removed and painful ones replace them. And, of course, we want to reverse this. We want to get rid of all those painful dishes: all those difficult problems we now have to deal with and all those agonising thoughts, feelings and memories. We want to sweep them off the table and bring back all those precious items we've lost. But, unfortunately, we aren't able to do that. So what can we do?

Well, this is where values come in handy. You can think of your values as what you want to bring to the table of life. Do you want to bring love, courage, kindness? Do you want to bring playfulness, openness, curiosity? Do you want to bring honesty, humour, helpfulness? You can bring these things to the table through your words, actions and gestures. You can't magically change what life has dished out for you — but you can add to what's there upon the table; and, as you do that, the dishes already there will transform.

You've already experienced this in Part 1 of the book. Life served up many painful thoughts, feelings, and memories — and what you brought to the table was kindness, caring and compassion. Do those words — kindness, caring, compassion — describe how, deep in your heart, you want to treat yourself and others? If so, you can think of them as 'values'.

Values versus goals

Values are radically different to goals. And if that statement confuses you, believe me, you're not alone; it confuses almost everyone. This is because we live in a goal-focused society, not a values-focused one. Indeed, often when people use the word 'values' they are actually talking about 'rules' or 'goals' instead. So let me clarify the difference. Values describe *how you want to behave*, while goals describe *what you want to get*. If you want to get a great job, buy a big house, find a partner, get married or have kids, those are all goals. They can all potentially be ticked off the 'to do' list: 'Goal achieved!' Values, in contrast, are how you want to behave every step of the way as you move towards your goals; how you want to behave when you achieve your goals; and how you want to behave when you *don't* achieve your goals!

For example, if your values are to be loving, kind and caring, then you can behave in these ways right now and forever — even if you never achieve the goal of finding a partner or having kids. (And, of course, some people do achieve those goals of having a partner and kids, but neglect to be kind, loving and caring.) Similarly, if in the workplace your values are to be productive, efficient, sociable, attentive and responsible, you can behave in these ways right now even if your job 'totally sucks'. (And some people do have a great job but neglect all those aforementioned values.)

Now, suppose you want to be loved or respected. Are those values? No, they are goals! They are all about trying to get something — in this case trying to get love or respect from others. Your values are how *you* want to behave as you pursue those goals, regardless of whether you achieve them or not. If you want to be loving or respectful, those *are* values; they are desired qualities of behaviour and you can act lovingly or respectfully to yourself or to others whenever you choose to. But to be loved or respected are goals (or some people call them 'needs') and they are out of our control; we can't make someone love us or respect us. In fact, the more we try to make someone love us or respect us, the less likely they are to do so! But if we act lovingly and respectfully towards ourselves and others, there's a good chance we will be loved and respected in return. (No guarantees, of course.)

Values and goals are both important — but we do need to keep in mind their differences, as we use them in different ways. The easiest way to remember the difference is: goals describe what I want to have, get or achieve; values describe how I want to treat myself, others or the world around me. And what has all this got to do with the reality slap? Well, once we have regrouped — through dropping anchor and self-compassion — the next step is to take action; to stand for something in the face of all our pain. (There is no fulfilment to be found in giving up on life — although, at times, most of us do.) So when life asks us the question: 'What will you stand for in the face of this great suffering?' we can find the answer in our values: 'I will stand for being the sort of person I want to be; I will stand for acting on what matters, deep in my heart.' And through this response we give ourselves something to live for; we give ourselves a cause or a purpose. We literally give our life meaning.

If this still doesn't make much sense to you, or you get the concept but you're not quite sure what your own values actually are ... then yes, you guessed it, that's normal. When I first start talking to people about meaning, purpose or values, they often become anxious, confused or go blank. So I take them through a couple of exercises to help them get the hang of it. The first one involves extracting the 'hidden wisdom' that gets buried beneath harsh self-judgment.

How's your mind trying to help?

Begin this exercise by taking a few moments to drop anchor.

Now recall some harsh self-judgments your mind keeps telling you.

Take a moment to name this story or pattern: perhaps 'Self-judgment', or 'The "Not Good Enough" story' or 'The inner critic'?

Now consider, when your mind keeps churning out these judgments, how's it trying to help?

Is it trying to help you learn from the past?

Is it trying to solve a problem, prepare you for something or make a plan?

Is it trying to save you from, protect you from, or prepare you for something in the future?

Is it connecting you with someone or something that matters?

Is it reminding you to take care of yourself or someone else?

What's it trying to help you do differently or better?

What personal qualities is it trying to bring out in you?

Natalie's mind had been really getting stuck, calling her a 'bad mother' in a hundred and one different ways. The morning her son died they'd had a heated row and she'd said some harsh words to him, calling him selfish and lazy. Those were the last words she ever spoke to him. She'd had various versions of the 'Bad Mother' story for many years, but now her mind was really doing a hatchet-job — replaying the entire back-catalogue of all the times she'd let her son down or treated him unkindly. She'd been dropping anchor, naming the story, making room, practising kind self-talk and the kind hand exercise, as well as doing her regular grieving rituals, and this had all been very helpful — but still her mind kept mercilessly beating her up.

As I took Natalie through the reflections above, she came up with some interesting answers. Obviously her mind was connecting her with her deep, deep love for her son, and wanting her to be 'a good mother' instead of a 'bad' one. 'So, according to your mind,' I asked, 'What are the personal qualities of a "good mother"?' With a bit of prompting, Natalie identified qualities such as loving, kind, forgiving, supportive, reliable. 'And those things are important to you? Deep in your heart, that's the sort of mother you want to be?'

'Yes!' she cried. 'But it's too late for that! He's dead.'

Through reflecting on the questions above, Natalie had tapped into some very important values. And, of course, she was right. Her son was dead, and there was no way to go back and change the past.

So I asked her: 'These values of yours — being loving, kind, forgiving, supportive, reliable — are they only for that one relationship, with Richard? Or are there other people in your life that you'd like to treat that way?'

'Of course there are,' she replied. 'My husband, my daughter, my friends, my parents …'

'So maybe this is what your mind is trying to help you with? To bring more of those values into your other relationships? Obviously that won't bring Richard back or change the past or get rid of your pain — but could there be something in it that's meaningful for you?' A glimmer of hope flickered across Natalie's face.

With Rada, the process was trickier. Because of her chronic illness (fibromyalgia), Rada had given up on many activities she had previously enjoyed, such as Latin dancing and aerobics — but her greatest loss was a rather unusual pastime. Rada loved to spend her weekends making abstract sculptures out of wood, clay and steel. (She had tried to make a living from her work but hadn't been successful.) Unfortunately, though, sculpting is physically strenuous, and the pain in Rada's arms, back and neck made it all but impossible. Because of this, Rada's mind kept calling her 'pathetic', 'weak', 'useless' and 'worthless'.

'I can't see how my mind is trying to help me,' she said.

We'd spoken before about the two ways to motivate a donkey — carrot and stick — so I said, 'I think your mind is using the big stick method — beating you up to try to get you to do something. What do you think it wants you to do?'

'To start dancing and sculpting and doing all the things I used to do.'

'Yes, I think so too.'

'But I can't do those things anymore!' cried Rada.

'That's right. At least for now, you can't. So, although your mind wants to help — it's actually getting in the way. First, it's using the big stick; and second, it's trying to push you into doing things that aren't currently realistic. So, how about you put down the stick and let's look at what *is* realistic for you to do, given the limitations imposed by your health.'

Rada agreed to do this, so our next step was to tease out the values underlying activities such as dancing and sculpting. I wanted to help her see that although she couldn't currently do those activities, she could still live the values that underpinned them. So I asked her: 'I'm wondering, if someone wanted to really get into sculpting — to enjoy it, appreciate it, do it well — what qualities do you think would help them to do that?'

'Errm, well — I guess dedication ... trying new things ... focus ... persistence ... creativity ... striving to grow or improve ... being real ... allowing yourself to make mistakes and learn from them.'

'And are those qualities important to you? Do they describe how you like to sculpt?'

'Yes! But I can't do it anymore!'

'Yes, and of course, that's very painful.' At this point, Rada burst into tears, flooding with sadness and anger; so we dropped anchor and practised the kind hands exercise. (As we do the painful work of rebuilding, we can expect emotional storms to keep blowing up, so it's important to keep using all the mindfulness and self-compassion skills we covered in Part 1.) After the exercise, we returned to the discussion. 'What you've been describing there — persistence, creativity, dedication, focus, growth, and so on — sound like important values.'

'Yes,' said Rada. 'They are.'

'So I'm wondering, are these values only for that one activity, sculpting? Or are there other activities in your life — activities you can do today even with all the limitations imposed by your illness — where you could bring some of these values into play? Obviously that wouldn't be the same as sculpting, and nor would it get rid of your pain. But I'm wondering, could there be something in it that's meaningful for you?'

Rada paused for a long time, thinking very carefully. Then, ever so slowly she nodded her head.

If you didn't actually do the 'How's your mind trying to help?' exercise, or you zipped through it quickly without actively reflecting on the questions, please go back and take your time with it (p. 137), and see if you can dig out some values.

And, if your mind is a bit like Rada's, trying to push you into doing something that's currently unrealistic or impossible, then find out the values underpinning that activity. A good way to do this is to ask yourself: 'If someone wanted to enjoy, appreciate or do this activity well, what personal qualities would help them to do so?'

You may recall in Chapter 6 I mentioned that many people question themselves — 'Who am I?' — after a major loss. 'Who am I without my job?', 'Who am I without a partner?', 'Who am I without my health?', 'Who am I without my parents?', 'Who am I without a child?' If your mind has been doing this, then it's basically trying to help you think deeply about what sort of person you want to be, what values you want to live by, what you want to stand for in the face of your loss. Hopefully the exercises in this chapter will help you to answer those questions.

Remember, our aim at this point is simply to get a sense of what our values are. In the next chapter, we're going to look at how to translate them into actions (and you'll find out what Natalie and Rada did next). So to get some more clarity about your values, here's another exercise called 'Connect and reflect'. (This was inspired by a similar exercise called 'The sweet spot', created by one of my mentors, Kelly Wilson.) I invite you to try it.

Connect and reflect

Part 1: Connect

Begin this exercise by taking a few moments to drop anchor.

Now think of someone who is active *in your life today*; someone you care about, someone you see regularly; someone with whom you like to spend quality time. And remember a recent time when you were with each other, doing some sort of activity you really like.

Make this memory as vivid as possible, as if it is happening here and now.

Relive it. Feel it emotionally.

Look out from behind your own eyes onto the scene: Notice where you are … Time of day? Indoors or outdoors? Weather? Scenery? Temperature? What's the air like? What can you see? What can you hear? What can you touch … taste … smell?

Notice the other person: What does he or she look like? What is he or she saying or doing? What's her tone of voice, the expression on his face, her body posture, the way he is moving?

In this memory, what are you thinking? And feeling? And doing? What are you doing with your arms … legs … mouth? Are you moving or still? Get into your body (in this memory); what does it feel like?

See if you can tap into the emotion of this memory; what does it *feel* like? Drink it in and let it flow through you; open up and make room for it. And you may well find as you do this, that you encounter some sadness, longing or regret. This is hardly surprising, because whatever we hold precious will usually bring us pain. So as you engage with this memory, be open and make room for all that arises: the pleasure *and* the pain.

Savour the moment. Make the most of it. Really appreciate it.

So how did you find that? Did you find it enjoyable? Did sadness or other painful emotions arise? If so, did you open up and make room for them, and practise self-compassion? That was actually just the first part of the exercise. The second part is to go back into that memory, take a good look at yourself ... and reflect.

Connect and reflect

Part 2: Reflect

Now step back and look at the memory as if you're watching it on a TV screen.

Focus on yourself. What are you saying and doing? How are you interacting with the other person? How are you treating him or her? How are you responding to him or her?

What qualities are you showing in this memory? For example, are you being open, engaged, interested, loving, kind, fun-loving, playful, connected, appreciative, honest, real, courageous, intimate?

What does this remind you about the sort of person you want to be?

What does this tell you about the way you want to treat yourself and others?

What does this highlight about the sort of relationships you want to build, and how you want to spend your time?

I'm guessing that in the 'connect and reflect' exercise you remembered a deep connection with someone. Now consider for a moment: in that memory, what are you bringing to the table? For example, are you contributing love, enthusiasm, curiosity, openness, attentiveness, appreciation, gratitude, sensuality, kindness, interest, playfulness, humour, warmth, affection, tenderness, honesty, trust?

Come up with three or four words that best describe the qualities of your behaviour in that memory. Now consider: are those qualities you *want* to bring to life's table? Are those qualities you *want* to bring into your relationships, through your words, gestures, deeds and actions? If so, then these too are your values.

Okay, now let's do one last exercise.

Looking back six months from now

Begin this exercise by taking a few moments to drop anchor. Now imagine that six months from now you are looking back on your life today, thinking about how you responded to your reality slap. From that perspective, answer some or all of these questions. (Please don't rush this. Take your time; really think about it.)

What did you stand for in the face of that reality slap?

How did you treat yourself as you went through it?

How did you treat the people you care about as you went through it?

> As you dealt with all the difficulties, what qualities did you bring to life's table?

I hope you're starting to get a sense now of at least some of your values. Sometimes our minds can make this process very hard for us: 'How do I know if these are my *real* values? Am I just picking them because I think I *should* have these as my values?' and so on. When you notice your mind doing that trick, name it: 'Ah, here's my mind over-analysing', 'I'm having thoughts of self-doubt', 'I'm noticing double-guessing'. Instead of getting caught up in 'analysis paralysis', pick a few values to play around with and notice what happens. When you start using these values in the manner that we discuss in the next chapter, you'll learn a lot about yourself — and usually it will rapidly become clear whether or not you've found your 'real' values.

Values, relationships and meaning

Suppose we think of our life as a huge and complex network of relationships. When I use the term 'relationship' I mean the way we interact with anyone or anything. In this sense of the word, we have relationships with ourselves; relationships with our thoughts and feelings and memories; relationships with our physical body; relationships with our family, friends and neighbours; relationships with our work and our leisure; relationships with our physical environment; and relationships with a vast number of inanimate objects such as our phone, our computer, the food we eat, the water we drink, the bed we sleep on, the place we live in and so on.

Rebuilding our life involves looking at the relationships we have and doing what we can to make them as healthy as possible. Sometimes we might buy into unhelpful stories such as 'Life has no meaning', 'I don't know what to do with my life' or 'Is this all there is?' But all we need to do, in any moment, to infuse our life with a sense of meaning and purpose is to choose a relationship that matters — with anyone or anything — and do something to make it better, healthier or more fulfilling. How do we that? By noticing what life is serving up in this moment, and bringing our values to the table.

For example, if there is somebody in your life who is toxic, abusive, hurtful, uncaring or heartless, you might choose to bring to the table qualities such as assertiveness, courage, fairness, self-respect, self-protection, self-support. Guided by these values you protect and look after yourself and actively reduce or stop the damage done by the other person. (This could involve restricting contact with them or even cutting them out of your life altogether.) Similarly, if there's an activity in your life that is self-defeating (e.g. withdrawing from or fighting with your loved ones), or a substance you partake of that is toxic in excess (e.g. tobacco, alcohol, junk food), then you might choose to bring to the table qualities such as self-awareness and self-care to actively break that pattern.

If there's somebody in your life who is warm and caring, then you might choose to bring qualities to the table such as appreciation, gratitude, love, kindness and trust. If there's an activity in your life that enriches or enhances it (such as connecting with your loved ones, having fun, listening to music, reading books, pursuing your hobbies or interests) then you might choose to bring qualities to the table such as being attentive, focused, interested, open, curious, engaged or appreciative.

Many self-help approaches focus on goals: on what we want to get from life and our relationships. Our values give rise to a very different attitude: they help us to look at what we want to actively contribute to life; what we want to give to our relationships. We will look at goals later, because they are very important; we're not going to pretend we don't need or want anything in life. But, for now, let's keep the focus on values and consider what happens when we actively bring them to the table. For example, consider your relationship with this book. As you read, are you bringing in qualities of openness, enthusiasm, curiosity, focusing, engaging? And does that make a difference? Have you ever had a relationship with a book where you *didn't* bring in qualities such as enthusiasm, curiosity, focusing, engaging? If so, was it rewarding and fulfilling — or did it feel like a waste of your time?

For another example, let's go back to the connect and reflect exercise. In that moment, you were contributing qualities that actively enhanced the relationship. How often do all of us contribute very different qualities — such as aggression, unkindness, unfairness, disinterest or disengagement — to our relationships with the people we love the most? And what happens to a relationship when that's what we bring to the table?

For one final example, let's go back to Part 1 of this book. What happens to our relationship with ourselves when we contribute qualities such as being harsh, unkind, judgmental or uncaring? And what happens when we bring in different qualities, such as kindness and caring?

The great thing about knowing our values is that we can *instantly* use them to make our life more meaningful. We don't have to wait until we find some noble cause or life mission; we can simply bring our values into any relationship — with anyone or anything — here and now. In the next chapter, we'll look at how to do that, but in the meantime let's finish with something to reflect on: a quote from the Canadian poet, Henry Drummond.

66 You will find, as you look back upon your life, that the moments when you have really lived are the moments when you have done things in the spirit of love."

14

ONE SMALL STEP

Have you ever heard this saying: 'It's the thought that counts'?
Let's think about this for a moment. Which means more
to you: when someone has a thought about buying you a birthday
present, or when they actually go out and buy you one? Which of
these will get you into trouble with the law: if you have thoughts about
committing a crime, or if you actually go out and commit one? Which
will count the most to your children: if you think about being a loving
and supportive parent, or if you actually are loving and supportive?
No child has ever said: 'What I really admired about my dad was
that although he was totally selfish and was never there for me when
I needed him, he often *thought* about being more caring and giving.'

So, let's face it: it's our actions that count, not our thoughts. And
it's just as well, or we'd all be in a lot of trouble. Think of all those
angry, vengeful thoughts you've had in your life; of all those times
you've thought of doing something to hurt another person, such as
yelling offensive insults or saying nasty put-downs, or committing
acts of revenge. And have you ever had thoughts about leaving your

partner, or quitting your job, or running away from your life? We all have plenty of thoughts that we would be embarrassed to admit to in public; so what state would our lives be in if these thoughts *really did* count more than our actions?

We create our life through our actions, not through our thoughts. One of my current clients has been seriously thinking about quitting his dull, tedious, undemanding job and retraining as a psychologist. The problem is, he's been thinking about it seriously for over ten years — and he still hasn't taken any action! And isn't he a bit like you and me? Most of us spend far too much time thinking about what we want to do with our time on this planet, but nowhere near enough time actually doing it.

Of course, usually when we say, 'It's the thought that counts', it serves a specific purpose: we are trying to make somebody else feel better. We suspect they are feeling bad because they haven't followed through on something they considered important (such as buying that birthday present), and we want to let them off the hook. So next time you're in this situation, why not say something that serves the same purpose, but is a bit more genuine and compassionate, like: 'Ah, well. You're only human. I do things like that too. Really, it's no big deal.'

And next time you're *thinking* about an important or meaningful area of your life, why not ask yourself these questions: 'What's a tiny step I could take? What's the smallest, easiest, simplest action I could do to make a difference in this part of my life?' After all, when it comes to creating the life you want, even the tiniest actions count for more than many hundreds of hours of thinking.

This is where our values can really help us. We can ask ourselves two simple questions:

- What relationship matters most in this moment?
- What do I want to bring to the table?

Let's look at a few examples to tease this out. Suppose the relationship that matters most right now is with your body; could you bring openness and curiosity to the table? Could you notice what your body is doing? How is it moving? Where is it tense and where is it relaxed? Where is it strong and where is it weak? What makes it function better and what makes it worse? Could you bring in some kindness and caring for your body — through stretching, or exercise, or eating well, or sleeping well, or giving it a rest, or teaching it a new skill, or taking it for a walk in the park?

And, if the most important relationship is with your mind, could you again bring openness and curiosity to the table? Notice what your mind is up to. Is it doing something useful? Is it fantasising, remembering, worrying, pondering or planning? If you wanted to be caring and helpful, could you give your mind a rest? Or could you teach it a new skill? Or could you introduce it to something interesting like some new books, music or movies?

And, if the most important relationship in this moment is with your art, or your sport, or your hobby, or your work, or your study, then what happens when you bring interest and attentiveness to the table; when you immerse your full attention in the task; when you give it your enthusiasm, curiosity, courage, creativity, care, consideration or patience?

And, if this relationship happens to be with a person, then the same question applies, regardless of whether that person is your partner, child, parent, friend, neighbour, teacher, student, mentor, customer, employer or co-worker. What do you want to bring to the table? Do you want to be engaged, curious, attentive, open, caring — or disengaged, uninterested, inattentive, closed off, uncaring? If the former, there are ways you can instantly do this. You might pay more attention to their face, their tone of voice, their body posture, or the words that they are saying. You might be curious about their emotions, their thoughts, or their beliefs, attitudes and assumptions. You might try to understand their world and their needs, or do small acts of kindness and caring.

Of course, if this other person is treating you badly you'll need to shift your priorities within this relationship. First and foremost, you'll need to take care of and contribute to *your own* health and wellbeing; to do what is necessary to protect and look after yourself and meet your own needs. And, if the bad treatment persists, you may well wish to consider ending the relationship. (Obviously this is not always possible — but, even if it is, it might not be the best option, for example, if you're caring for a loved one who has some sort of illness that leads them to be abusive.) Either way, while the relationship persists, your priority should be on caring for yourself within it.

In the last chapter, you connected with your values. The challenge now is to translate them into actions. What can you say — silently to yourself or out loud to others — that brings your values to the table? What can you do with your arms and your legs, your hands and your feet, the expressions on your face, the postures of your body, the tone of your voice that puts your values into play?

One brick at a time

Last chapter we talked about how walls are built one brick at a time. It's wise to take this same step-by-step approach to rebuilding our life after loss, so we don't get overwhelmed. With this in mind, think of your life in terms of four overarching domains: work and education; family and friends; play and leisure; and health and wellbeing. Each week, I recommend you pick *just one* of these four domains to actively work on.

The work and education domain includes paid work, volunteer work, or any area of study, training or learning. Family and friends can include your children, parents, partner, relatives, friends and anyone else you care deeply about. Play and leisure includes your hobbies, interests, creative pursuits, sports that you play or follow, and anything you like to do for rest or relaxation. Health and wellbeing includes anything you do to actively contribute to your physical, emotional, spiritual or psychological health and wellbeing. (Of course, these domains all overlap with each other — they're not really separate at all. This is just a convenient way of looking at different aspects of your life. The good news is, because of the interconnectedness of these domains, there's often a domino effect: while you're working on one, it impacts positively another.)

Once you've chosen a domain to work on, pick two or three values you want to bring to the table. (If you really want to, you can choose up to four or five values but more than that gets hard to remember.) Then consider how you might actively live those values within that domain. What new activities might you start? How might you modify activities you're already doing? What actions might you take? What words might you say? How might you treat yourself, others or the world around you?

Antonio chose to work first of all in the family and friends domain, with a special focus on his relationship with Cathy. And he chose the values of kindness, understanding and openness. He stopped drinking heavily, zoning out in front of the TV, picking fights. He started listening to her with genuine kindness, holding her when she cried, going for a long walk with her in the evenings, during which they would both talk openly and honestly about their grief. This didn't take away Antonio's grief and suffering; but it did give him a sense of being true to himself, of being the sort of partner he really wanted to be, deep in his heart.

Shanti also chose the family and friends domain, and the values of courage, openness and honesty. One by one, she started to reconnect with her friends and family; this was very courageous, in and of itself, as it brought up huge feelings of shame and anxiety. She also chose to be honest and open about those feelings rather than hide them away and put on a happy face. To her surprise, she found most of her loved ones were kind and understanding. Unfortunately, some of them were inept at providing the support she needed — and her mother, appallingly, blamed Shanti for the affair: 'If you'd been a better wife, he wouldn't have gone looking.' So Shanti also brought along her values of self-compassion and self-protection. She minimised time with her mother and treated herself kindly whenever her mother was toxic. Instead she spent most of her time with the people who could truly be there for her in a loving and nurturing way. This didn't get rid of her sadness, or her anger, or all those painful memories; but it did give her a sense of reclaiming her life.

Dave had lost his job, so not surprisingly the domain he chose first was work and education. The values he picked were patience, persistence and responsibility. He allocated 8 hours every day where he would either actively pursue the goal of finding a new job, or actively educate himself in skills and knowledge that would help him in that pursuit. The tedious tasks of writing a CV, searching for jobs, applying for jobs and going for interviews gave Dave ample opportunities to live his values. Each morning, as he prepared himself for all those unpleasant (and unpaid) tasks he needed to do, he'd drop anchor and repeat his values silently, like a mantra: 'Patience, persistence, responsibility'. This didn't make his tasks easy or fun; but it did give him a sense of empowerment. He had no power to escape all the discomfort and hassle that's involved in finding a new job. And he also had no power to ensure that he'd get the job he wanted. But he did have the power to choose his own attitude, to choose what he'd bring to the table in the face of his difficulties.

Natalie chose to focus on health and wellbeing. The values she picked were self-care and self-kindness. She practised the kind hands exercise every day and worked hard at unhooking from the 'Bad Mother' story. She'd lost a lot of weight since Richard's death and was now unhealthily thin. So, even though she still had no appetite, in the service of self-care, she started drinking protein shakes to increase her calorie intake. Of course, this could never bring her son back or diminish her agony at his loss. But it did give her a sense of establishing a little control amidst all the chaos. And it did help her to tap into those nurturing, caring instincts she'd always had as a mother.

Rada chose to focus on the domain of play and leisure, and to bring in the values of creativity, persistence and openness (openness to trying new things; openness to making mistakes and learning from them). She couldn't do sculpting or dancing, but she found other ways to bring those values to the table. For example, she experimented with her stretching and strengthening exercises, and ways of doing them in time to very slow, rhythmic, soothing music — like an ultra-slow-motion minimalist dance routine. A long way from Latin dancing, but nonetheless a way to live her values of creativity, openness and persistence (and make her physiotherapy routine a lot more interesting).

She also started a new creative activity that she hadn't done since high school: pencil drawing. It was nothing remotely like sculpting, and she had no 'natural talent' to draw upon; but it did give her the satisfaction of being creative and open to learning.

So, now, let's come back to you. I encourage you, for at least the next month, to pick one domain of life each week to focus on. (It can be the same domain every week, if you like; you don't have to change over if you prefer not to.) And pick two or three values (five at most) to play with, and start actively bringing them in to what you do.

And if you're not clear about what to do differently, then keep doing what you're doing — but now, as you do those activities, look for opportunities to 'flavour' them with your values. For example, let's suppose you choose the domain of family and friends, and the values of warmth and playfulness. When you're with your loved ones, look for opportunities to sprinkle a bit of warmth and kindness into the interaction through the words you say or the things you do, or even through the expression on your face and your tone of voice.

And as you flavour the moment with those values, also take the time to savour it. Actively notice and appreciate the difference it makes. Notice what it's like to behave the way you really want to, deep in your heart. What's it like for you? What's it like for the people you care about? Is life more meaningful, more fulfilling? Is this something you would like to do more? Flavour your moments with values and savour what happens when you do.

Flavouring and savouring

Whether you start doing new things — like Rada with her drawing, and Dave with his job-searching — or whether you keep on doing much the same as before, liberally sprinkle your values into your life.

One way to do this is with a simple drill that takes less than a minute. Once or twice a day, take a few moments to drop anchor, and think of two or three values that you want to bring to the table in the next few hours. (It may be the same two or three values every time, or you may prefer to change them.) Then, as you go through the day, look for opportunities to flavour your activities with those values.

And be flexible with this. You can sprinkle your values into other domains as well; you don't have to stick to the one you've chosen to focus on. Likewise, if there's an opportunity to sprinkle in some different values (i.e. different to the ones you chose in the morning) then please, don't hold back. Flavour your experiences with your values, and savour what happens when you do.

15

THE CHALLENGE FORMULA

You can't cross the sea merely by
standing and staring at the water.
— *Rabindranath Tagore*

Life is both kind and cruel; it doles out both wonder and dread in generous portions. In my years as a GP, I met many people who had suffered terribly in life. I saw children disfigured by fire and babies with fatal diseases. I saw strong capable adults reduced to invalids and brilliant minds wiped away by dementia. I saw bodies misshapen and deformed through all manner of injury — the victims of violence and disaster. I saw refugees from foreign lands, struggling to rebuild their lives after rape and torture, or to start again after losing most of their family. I saw the freshly bereaved, howling in their anguish; distraught mothers clutching their stillborn babies. I saw men with weeping sores and blistering skin, and women with broken bones and bleeding arteries. I saw the blind, the deaf and the paralysed, the seriously ill and the newly deceased.

And, in the midst of all this pain, I saw courage, kindness and compassion. I saw people reaching out and helping each other; families bonding through crisis; friends and neighbours holding each other's hands. I saw men and women facing death with dignity; love and affection pouring from broken hearts. I saw parents slowly rebuilding shattered lives; finding the strength within to persist and grow.

A terrible crisis can prompt us to open our hearts and search within, to reach inside and discover what we are made of. However, this may take a while. And this may vary from hour to hour, day to day, week to week. There'll likely be times when we want to give up on life — and we do. Times when it's all too much, and we just want to retreat.

This is only to be expected; it's what comes naturally. We use what methods we know to try to escape, anything from movies and music to drinking and drugs. And even if we escape for only a moment, the relief is huge. However, a life lived in retreat is not fulfilling. And if we spend our days in a constant fight with reality we will soon be exhausted. So if we want to thrive in the face of a huge reality slap, our best option is to open ourselves to life as it is in this moment, and stand for something that matters deep in our heart. To help us with this task, we can draw upon a strategy that I like to simply call …

The challenge formula

No matter how great the challenge we are facing, we are not powerless. We have choices. Even in the most difficult situations, we always have either two or three options:

1. Leave.

2. Stay and live by your values: do whatever you can to improve the situation, make room for the inevitable pain that goes with it and hold yourself kindly.

3. Stay and do things that either make no difference or make it worse.

Of course, option 1 — leave — isn't always available. For example, if you're in prison or a refugee camp, you can't just up and leave. If the situation is you've got a serious illness, or you've lost a loved one, you can't simply leave that situation; wherever you go, the problem goes with you. But at times, leaving the situation *is* an option — in which case, seriously consider it. For example, if you're in a toxic relationship, an awful job, a violent neighbourhood, consider: is your life likely to be richer, fuller, more meaningful if you leave that situation rather than stay?

Now if you can't leave, won't leave, or don't consider leaving to be the best option, then you are down to options 2 and 3. Unfortunately, for most of us option 3 comes quite naturally: *Stay and do things that either make no difference or make it worse.* In challenging situations, we easily get hooked by difficult thoughts and feelings and pulled into self-defeating patterns of behaviour which either keep us stuck or make things worse. We may turn to excessive use of drugs and alcohol, fighting with or withdrawing from loved ones, dropping out of important parts of life, or zillions of other self-defeating behaviours. (I know I've often fallen into these patterns, and I'm pretty sure you have too.)

So the path to a better life clearly lies in option 2: *Stay and live by your values, and do whatever you can to improve the situation.* And of course, you can't expect to feel happy when you're in a really difficult situation; you are guaranteed to have plenty of painful thoughts and feelings. So the second part of option 2 — *make room for the inevitable pain and hold yourself kindly* — is very relevant. That's why we spent so much time in Part 1 of this book on learning how to make room for painful thoughts, feelings and memories; how to take the impact and power out of them; how to allow them to be present without letting them jerk us around; and how to respond to our pain with genuine kindness.

The life of Nelson Mandela gives an excellent example of the challenge formula in action. For twenty-seven years, he was imprisoned by the South African government. Why? Because he dared to fight for freedom and democracy; to oppose apartheid, the official government policy of racial discrimination. Now option 1 of the formula was clearly out: he couldn't *leave* prison. So, mostly, he chose option 2. He made room for his painful feelings, and he lived according to his values: standing for freedom, equality and peace. For instance, during his first seventeen years in prison, on Robben Island, Mandela had to do hard labour in a lime quarry. But he turned the situation to his advantage. You see, Mandela knew that education was essential for equality and democracy, so he arranged illegal meetings in the tunnels of the quarry where the prisoners would teach and instruct each other. (Later this came to be known as 'Mandela University'.)

One of the most remarkable aspects of Mandela's story is that in 1985, after twenty-two years in prison, the South African government offered to release him — but he turned them down! Why? Because the condition for release was that he would have to remain silent; that he would refrain from speaking out against apartheid. For Mandela to do this, he would have had to go against his core values, so he chose to stay in prison instead. That meant *another five years in prison* before he was finally released without this condition! And yet, despite this huge reality slap, he was able to find fulfilment in standing for something: freedom, democracy and equality. Mandela's case is extraordinary, but the challenge formula applies to every one of us, no matter what our situation is. If we can't or won't leave, then we can stay and live by our values, do what we can to improve things, and make room for the pain that's inevitable.

In Chapter 1, I mentioned an ACT program that I wrote for the World Health Organization for use in refugee camps around the world. The program consists mostly of audio recordings; the refugees, in small groups, listen to them. The recordings explain ACT concepts and then ask the group members to do exercises similar to the ones in this book. The challenge formula comes in early on the very first session. The reality is, if you're in a refugee camp you can't just up and leave, so option 1 is out. But you do still have choices between options 2 and 3. For example, there are people who share the tent with you, and you can treat them with kindness, warmth and openness — or you can treat them with aggression, coldness or hostility. And the choices you make will alter your experience within that tent. And when you leave the tent, the same holds true. You can be kind and friendly to your neighbours in other tents, or distant and unfriendly. You can join in with community activities such as singing or prayer; or you can isolate yourself from them. The more you choose option 2 — *Stay and live by your values: do whatever you can to improve the situation, make room for the inevitable pain that goes with it and hold yourself kindly* — the better your quality of life within the camp.

Being realistic

When it comes to option 2, it's important to be realistic. If you're in prison or in a refugee camp, or suffering from a serious illness or injury, there are all sorts of things you can't do. And if you focus too much on what you *can't* do, that's a recipe for misery. Much wiser to focus on what you *can* do. Rada's mind kept pushing her to sculpt and dance when it wasn't realistic to do those things, and that made her all the more depressed. But when she focused on what she *could* do, living her values in other ways, her life was far more fulfilling.

Our minds often tell us about what we don't have or can't do — and that's normal. And we can't stop our minds from doing that, but we can unhook from it: 'Aha, here's the "Can't Do It" story', 'There's my mind reminding me of all the things I'm lacking', 'I'm noticing thoughts about what I can't do.' And we can acknowledge how painful it is, and open up and make room for those difficult feelings, and respond to ourselves with kindness. And we can come back to our values and act on them in the face of all our challenges.

I've focused so far mainly on small steps, small actions and small changes in behaviour. When we rebuild our lives after a reality slap, we do it mostly through these small changes. If we set big goals for ourselves it may backfire; all too often, we do not have the time, energy or other resources we need to achieve these goals, and it all gets too overwhelming and we give up. Small changes are much easier to make and sustain, and over time they often have dramatic effects. Sometimes, however, we do need to set goals for ourselves, and if so, it's important to make them realistic. To set goals effectively is quite a skill, and most of us are not naturally good at it. So if you'd like some help with this, go to Appendix C, which will guide you step by step through the process. And, of course, once you've set some goals, the next step is to take action!

We can never know in advance if we'll achieve our goals or not — but we *can* start taking action right away. And the moment we do, we will experience a sense of empowerment; a sense of embracing life and making the most of it, instead of letting it pass us by.

Willingness

When I present the challenge formula to my clients, most of them feel empowered: it helps them to realise they have choices. However, from time to time, someone has a strong negative reaction: usually a mixture of anger and anxiety. Why should this be? Usually because they find it too confronting. The challenge formula confronts us with the reality that we have choices and therefore we are responsible for how we act. There is short-term relief in option 3: in buying the story that's there's nothing we can do, so we may as well give up, stop trying. This can be a relief because it relieves us of responsibility. But any such relief does not last long. In the long term, this option drains the life from us. Our vitality lies only in taking a stand: in choosing options 1 or 2. However, we will only experience this vitality if we take our stand with a quality known as 'willingness'.

What does 'willingness' mean? Well, psychologist Hank Robb explains it as follows. Suppose you hand over $20 for a ticket to the movies. You can give the money resentfully or grudgingly, or you can give the money willingly, but either way you still have to hand over the money. And when you pay it willingly, the experience is far more fulfilling than if you do so resentfully.

So, when we take a stand, let's do so willingly. If we take this stand hooked by 'I have no choice', 'I hate having to do this', 'I shouldn't have to do this', 'This is my lot in life' or 'I have to do it; it's my duty', we will feel burdened, disempowered or drained. There is no 'have to', 'must', 'ought' or 'should' in a value; such words only turn our values into life-draining rules.

How do we distinguish rules from values? Well, rules can usually be identified by words such as 'right', 'wrong', 'good', 'bad', 'should', 'shouldn't', 'have to', 'must', 'ought', 'can't unless', 'shouldn't because' or 'won't until'. Rules tell you how to live your life: the right and wrong way of doing things. Values do *not* do this; values simply describe the qualities you wish to bring to your ongoing behaviour. So 'Thou shalt not kill' is a rule. It tells you what you should and shouldn't do; what is right and wrong. The values underneath this rule are caring and respect (for human life). If being loving is your value, this is obviously very different to a rule such as 'You *must* always be loving, no matter what!'. If being kind is your value, that's a world apart from a rule like 'You *should* be kind at all times, even when people are abusive to you'. If being efficient is your value, that's a long way from the rule, 'You *must* do it perfectly or there's no point.'

Of course, we can use our values to help set rules that guide us, but we do need to be clear that they are not one and the same thing. Values give us a sense of freedom because there are so many different ways in which we can act on them. In contrast, rules often give us a sense of restriction or obligation; they often weigh us down and limit our options. Suppose we help someone out because we're consciously in touch with our values: we wish to be kind and generous. Now compare this to helping someone out because we're hooked by rules: 'it's the right thing to do' or we 'should do it', we 'owe them' or we 'are obliged to'. The former approach tends to be freeing and energising; the latter is often restrictive, draining and burdensome.

So if you feel drained, burdened or resentful as you take a stand, pause for a moment and notice what unhelpful story has hooked you. Then name the story and drop anchor to help yourself unhook. After this, come back to your values and recognise that you *do* have a choice. You can *choose* to stand for something — or not. You certainly don't *have to*. The big question is, are you *willing* to? Ask yourself: 'Am I *willing* to take a stand in the face of this reality slap? Am I *willing* to make room for my pain and act on my values?'

16

THE PRISON OF RESENTMENT

Do you ever get caught up in resentment? Many of us do, especially after a major reality slap. We may resent others because they let us down, they treated us badly, they didn't care about us, they achieved more than us, they're 'better off' than us, or for dozens of other reasons. Resentment is a particularly sticky version of the 'Not Good Enough' story, a version heavily infused with anger, righteousness and a strong sense of injustice.

When we get hooked by resentment it almost always pulls us into self-defeating struggles. In Buddhism they say: 'Resentment is like grasping a red-hot coal in order to throw it at someone else.' In Alcoholics Anonymous (AA) they say: 'Resentment is like swallowing poison and hoping the other person dies.' What these sayings have in common is the idea that when we get hooked by resentment, all we do is hurt ourselves even more than we already are.

Resentment comes from the French word *resentir*, which means 'to feel again'. This makes sense: each time resentment hooks us we *feel again* our hurt, our anger, and our sense of unfairness or injustice.

The events that happened are now in the past, but as we dwell on them in the present we *feel again* all that pain. And as we stew in our anger and dissatisfaction, all our vitality seeps away.

A somewhat similar story is self-blame, which we can think of as resentment turned on ourselves. Again and again our minds remind us of all the things we did wrong, then we get angry and judge or punish ourselves. We *feel again* all our pain, regret, angst, disappointment and anxiety.

This does not alter the past in any way, nor does it enable us to learn and grow from our mistakes; all we achieve is to hurt ourselves more. And even though we know this logically and rationally, we still keep doing it.

Forgiveness

So what is the antidote to resentment and self-blame? It is 'forgiveness'. But not forgiveness as we commonly think of it. In the ACT model, forgiveness does *not* mean forgetting. Nor does it mean that what happened was okay, or excusable, or unimportant. And nor does it involve saying or doing anything to someone else.

To understand the ACT notion of forgiveness, let's consider the origin of the word. 'Forgive' is derived from two separate words: 'give' and 'before'. So in ACT, forgiveness simply means this: *giving* yourself back what life was like *before* resentment took over. At some point in the past — it may have been recent or a long time ago — something very painful happened. Either *you* did something that you now blame yourself for, or *others* did something that you now blame them for. And since that time, your mind has repeatedly pulled you back to those events, getting you to feel all the pain, again and again, along with all the blaming and judging and struggling.

So what was your life like *before* resentment took over? Were you getting on with life and making the most of it? Were you living in the present? Even if your life *wasn't* very good before resentment took over, at least you weren't lost in the choking smog of resentment and self-blame. So how about giving yourself back the clarity and freedom of life without all that smog? You see, in the ACT model forgiveness has nothing to do with anybody else; it is something you do purely for yourself. It's *giving* yourself a life free from the burden of resentment or self-blame.

How do we cultivate this type of forgiveness? You already have all the knowledge and skills you need. When our minds generate stories that tend to feed resentment or self-blame, our first steps are to notice them and name them. We could say to ourselves something like, 'I'm noticing my mind beating up on me' or 'I'm having a painful memory' or 'Here's my mind judging me' or 'I'm having thoughts about being bad'. At the same time, we can hold ourselves kindly. Whether we believe that we are at fault, or others are at fault, the undeniable fact is we are hurting. So let's be kind and compassionate and hold ourselves gently, make room for our feelings and get present.

We will often need to drop anchor repeatedly. Our mind will carry us off to those old events and we will have to bring ourselves back and get present: to engage and re-engage in the here and now. Then, once present, we can act in line with our values and infuse our ongoing action with a sense of purpose. We can then take a stand in the face of this reality gap.

For example, if we genuinely did do something 'wrong', 'bad' or 'careless' — and it's not just the mind being overly critical — then we could now take a stand to make amends. Michael, an alcoholic and Vietnam veteran, told me that in his case this was impossible:

he had killed several people in the war and there was no way to make amends for that. Well, it's hard to argue with that, so I didn't even try. Instead I said, 'Beating yourself up and drinking yourself into the grave isn't going to alter the past. And yes, of course you can't make amends to the dead; you can't do *anything* for the dead. But you *can* do something in the present that can contribute in meaningful ways to the *living*. If you waste your life away, then nothing good has come from those horrors of the past. But if you use your life to contribute to others, to make a difference in the world, then something good *has* come out of those horrors.'

For Michael, this was a revelation. It took him a lot of practice, but eventually he was able to unhook himself from those self-blaming stories and treat himself kindly. And over the space of nine months he joined an AA group, quit drinking and started volunteering for two charitable organisations: one for the homeless and the other for refugees. Now, this wasn't easy for him. It took a huge amount of hard work and he had to make room for enormous amounts of pain. But it paid off handsomely. Although he couldn't change the past, he found he could make a useful difference in the present — and as he did so, his life became far more fulfilling.

While most of us get entangled in self-blame at times, our stories are probably not as dramatic as Michael's; after all, most of us have never killed someone! However, that doesn't make our stories any less of a burden. The key thing is to practise being kind to yourself (even if your mind says you don't deserve it). It's often useful to say some kind words to yourself, such as: 'I'm a fallible human being. Like every other person on the planet, I make mistakes, I screw things up and I get things wrong. This is part of being human.' Then place a compassionate hand upon your body, breathe into the pain and acknowledge it hurts.

And remind yourself that self-punishment achieves nothing useful; vitality lies only in taking a stand. If there is something you can do to make amends, repair the damage or turn the situation around, then it makes sense to go ahead and do it. If there's nothing you *can* do along those lines (or if you're not yet *willing* to do it), then you can invest your energy in building the relationships you have: connecting, caring and contributing. To do this is an act of self-forgiveness.

But what if someone else did the 'bad stuff'? Well, we could respond in many different ways, depending on the specifics of the situation and the outcomes we are looking for. We might choose to take decisive action to ensure, as best we can, that something like this doesn't happen again: to take that person to court, or lodge a complaint against them, or cut off all contact with them. Or we might choose to learn new skills that equip us better for dealing with such people in the future; this could include anything from self-defence classes to assertiveness and communication skills, to attending a course on 'dealing with difficult people'. Or we might join organisations, sign petitions, go on marches, raise funds, support causes to change laws, improve society or make the world a better place. Or we might choose simply to 'put it behind us' and focus on rebuilding our life, here and now.

Forgiveness, then, consists of these four steps: drop anchor, unhook from the story, hold yourself kindly, and take a stand. And the beautiful thing about it is … it's never too late.

17

IT'S NEVER TOO LATE

I never would have believed it possible — not in a million years. My dad was a fairly typical guy for his generation. He looked after his kids in the traditional ways: he worked hard to pay the bills and ensured that his six children all had food and clothes, a roof over their head and a good education. He was very kind and loving in his own way. And, like most men of his generation (and many men of my own), he was terrified of intimacy. And by intimacy, I don't mean having sex; I mean emotional and psychological intimacy.

To be emotionally and psychologically intimate with another human requires two things:

1. You need to open up and be real; to 'let the other person in'; to share your true thoughts and feelings instead of hiding them away.

2. You need to create a space for the other person to do likewise; to be warm, open and accepting enough that they too can be real and open with you.

My dad never wanted to talk about anything deeply personal. He liked to make intellectual small talk: to exchange facts, figures and ideas; to discuss movies and books and science. This was all well and good — we had plenty of enjoyable conversations — but it meant that I never got to know him very well. I never got to know about the feelings he struggled with, his hopes and dreams, his setbacks and failures, his most important life experiences and what he learned from them. I never got to know what made him frightened or angry or insecure or sad or guilty. I knew virtually nothing of his interior world.

At the age of seventy-eight he developed lung cancer, but he didn't tell me. So, knowing nothing of his diagnosis, I went on a six-week trip overseas. Before I left, my dad had a full head of thick white hair, but when I got back he was totally bald. He didn't tell me that all his hair had fallen out due to the chemotherapy he'd been having. Instead, he told me he'd shaved off his hair because it was fashionable and he thought it made him look younger. And I believed him.

Of course, as he got sicker and frailer, the true story emerged. But even then, he didn't want to talk about his cancer, or the treatment, or his fears. And every time I tried to talk about it, he changed the subject or went quiet.

Not knowing how long he would live, I tried to tell him what he meant to me as a father: how much I loved him, the role he had played in my life, the ways he had inspired me, the most useful things he had taught me and the fondest memories I had of him. But he was so uncomfortable with such conversations, especially as my eyes would usually brim with tears, that he would end them almost as soon as they started.

Miraculously, he recovered from the cancer. I hoped this brush with death would help him to open up a little, but I was disappointed. He remained as closed off as he'd always been, if not more so.

Three years later, at the age of eighty-one, he had a heart attack. He had major blockages in several coronary arteries and he required open-heart surgery. The operation carried a significant risk of mortality. Talking to him shortly before the operation, I tried once again to share with him what he meant to me as a father. As usual, tears welled up in my eyes — tears of both love and sadness — and he instantly closed off. He turned away and said, in a stern voice, 'Hush now. And wipe away those tears.'

Dad survived the operation, but it knocked him around. He had one complication after another and spent most of the next year in hospital. Towards the end of that year, he became increasingly weak and more and more demoralised. And yet, he still would not allow me to talk to him on an intimate level. Eventually, he decided he had had enough of life and chose to stop all his medication. Being a doctor himself, he knew exactly what this meant: effectively he was killing himself. Once medication ceased, he knew full well he would have only a few days to live. And, even knowing this, he still refused to let me tell him how much I loved him and what he meant to me.

In the last hours of his life, Dad started hallucinating. But in between the hallucinations, he had lucid periods, where for several minutes at a time he would be fully conscious, mentally alert and in touch with reality. During one of these periods, I tried one last time to tell him what he meant to me and how much I loved him. I was a blubbering mess, tears streaming down my face and snot bubbling out of my nose. And to my utter amazement, Dad turned and looked deep into my eyes. His face lit up with a radiant smile, full of kindness and compassion, and he took my hands in his and he listened intently to everything I had to say, never once turning away or interrupting.

After I had finished sobbing and blowing my nose and telling him everything I'd been wanting to tell him for years, he said, in a voice full of tenderness and love, 'Thank you.' And then he added, 'I love you, too.'

I tell this story to make two key points, both of them vital to cover before we end this section. The first is that small changes can have a profound impact. My dad did not transform his personality; all he did was make one small change: he made the effort to stay present and open. And even though the whole episode was over within a few minutes, that one small change gave rise to a beautiful and loving experience that I'll remember fondly until the day I die.

Our society bombards us with the notion that if we wish to have a better life, we have to dramatically overhaul every part of it, or radically transform our personality, or fundamentally alter the way we think (or even do all three!). But the problem is, when we buy into these notions, it doesn't usually help us; commonly, all that happens is we end up placing enormous pressure on ourselves. We push ourselves harder and harder to be different and 'better' than what we are — and we beat ourselves up for not meeting our own expectations. Sadly, rather than raising us up, this just brings us down.

So why not lighten the load? Why not take the pressure off ourselves? Rome wasn't built in a day, and neither was a rich and meaningful life. Why not relax a little? Take baby steps. Go slow. And remember the moral of Aesop's much-loved tale of *The Crow and the Pitcher*: 'Little by little does the trick.'

Trying to make huge changes in a short space of time is almost always a recipe for failure. Occasionally we might manage it, but far more commonly we don't. However, small changes, over time, can make an enormous difference. To quote Archbishop Desmond Tutu: 'Do your little bit of good where you are; it's those little bits of good put together that overwhelm the world.'

The second important point of this story is that it's never too late to start making these little changes. Of course, your mind may not agree with that. The human mind is a bit like a 'reason-giving machine': it is brilliant at coming up with all sorts of reasons why we can't change, shouldn't change or shouldn't have to change, and one of its favourites is this: 'It's too late! I can't change now. That's the way I am. That's the way I've always been.' But we don't have to buy into such thoughts. Instead of seeing ourselves as 'carved in stone', we can acknowledge that we have a never-ending capacity to learn and grow and act and think differently. All we need to do is tune into our hearts and ask ourselves: 'What's one tiny change I could make? What's one tiny thing I could say or do differently, that's more in line with the person I want to be?'

I wish my dad had made his change a bit earlier, instead of waiting until he was on his deathbed. But I am so grateful for his precious parting gift: he opened up, stayed present, and allowed me to share my true feelings with him. And he did this *willingly*. It is such a beautiful memory: both heart-warming and heart-rending at the same time. And it's a powerful reminder that as long as we're still breathing, it's never too late to do something meaningful.

18

BREAKING BAD HABITS

Mark Twain once said: 'To cease smoking is the easiest thing in the world. I know because I've done it a thousand times.' Even if we've never smoked, most of us can relate to the witty observation of this famous author. How often have you said, 'I'm never going to do that again!' and, sure enough, the next day, you do it again? How often have you thought, 'Next time, I'm going to handle this differently?' And next time comes around, and shock horror: you end up doing the same old thing!

The truth is, even when life's going well it's easy to fall into 'bad habits'. But when we're coping with a big reality slap, our tendency to do so is much greater. By 'bad habits', I mean the patterns of behaviour that constitute option 3 of the challenge formula: *Stay and do things that either make no difference or make it worse.* This can include anything from excessive use of drugs and alcohol to withdrawal from friends and family; from aggression and conflict to avoiding important tasks or physical exercise.

We all have many 'bad habits' and it would be foolhardy to try to break all of them. As I've said in other chapters, the trick to success is making small changes: lay one brick at a time. If you try to work on several 'bad habits' at once you're likely to get overwhelmed and give up. However, if there is *one* bad habit that you consider really important to work on, the good news is you now have all the skills you need to break it. Of course, it will take time, and effort, and commitment. To quote Mark Twain again: 'Habit is habit, and not to be flung out of the window by any man, but coaxed downstairs a step at a time.' But, if it's important to you, you *can* do it.

Changing patterns of behaviour

There are six questions to answer when changing a self-defeating pattern of behaviour:

1. What am I doing?
2. What triggers it?
3. What are the payoffs?
4. What are the costs?
5. What's the alternative?
6. What skills can I use?

Let's explore these one at a time.

1. What am I doing?

The first step in changing a problematic pattern of behaviour is to specify what it involves: what are you actually saying and doing? For example, the term 'procrastinating' doesn't specify what you *are* doing; it refers to what you're *not* doing. If you're procrastinating on some important task or activity, then specify what you are doing instead:

are you playing computer games, reading the news, staring at the wall, eating snacks, stroking the dog, lying in bed?

If the habit is 'avoiding friends', what does this actually involve you saying and doing? Are you ignoring text messages, declining invitations, making excuses, cancelling social events at the last minute?

Antonio initially said that his problematic behaviour was 'drinking too much'. So I asked him to be more specific: 'How much are you actually drinking?' It turned out to be 'seven or eight bottles of beer a night'.

2. What triggers it?

It's important to identify what triggers the behaviour in question: what situations, thoughts and feelings 'set it off'? When and where does it tend to happen? Are there particular people, places, situations, events that tend to trigger it? What thoughts, feelings, memories, emotions, sensations or urges show up immediately before you start doing it? (If you're not sure what thoughts and feelings trigger your behaviour, best to keep a diary. Write down when and where you do it and see if you can identify what you were feeling and thinking just before you started.)

Antonio identified that the triggering situation was returning home after work. His triggering thoughts and feelings were anxiety, guilt, tightness in his chest, knots in his stomach, painful memories of Sophia, thoughts like, 'Oh no. Here we go again; another tense evening' … and, of course, urges to drink beer.

3. What are the payoffs?

Any type of behaviour has both payoffs (outcomes that convey some sort of benefit) and costs (outcomes that are in some way detrimental).

It's not absolutely essential to know what the payoffs are, but it's often helpful to identify them. Why? Because it gives you insight into why you keep doing it. If there were no payoffs, you'd stop doing the behaviour; so it's good to know what you're getting out of it. Basically the payoffs boil down to this:

- You get away from something you don't want.

- You get access to something you do want.

What follows are some of the most common payoffs for 'bad habits'.

- We get to escape or avoid people, places, situations or events that we find challenging.

- We get to escape or avoid unwanted thoughts, feelings, memories, sensations or urges.

- We feel better.

- We get our needs met.

- We gain attention.

- We look good (to others or to ourselves).

- We feel like we are right (and others are wrong).

- We feel like we are successfully following important rules.

- We feel like we are working hard on our problems.

- We feel like we are making sense (of life, the world, ourselves, others etc.).

Antonio was readily able to see that drinking beer helped him to a) escape difficult thoughts and feelings, and b) make him feel more relaxed. If you can't figure out the payoffs of your behaviour, that's okay. You don't need to know them in order to change it; it's useful, but not essential.

4. What are the costs?

Presumably you're already aware of some costs to this behaviour or you wouldn't be wanting to change it. However, it's worth spending a bit of time reflecting more deeply on this issue. What does this behaviour cost you in terms of health, wellbeing, vitality, relationships, money, wasted time, missed opportunities? What meaningful or valuable things do you lose or miss out on when you do this? And what do you get that you don't want? (This is not an excuse to start beating yourself up. If your mind pulls out that big stick and starts whacking you around with the 'Not Good Enough' story, drop anchor, unhook, and hold yourself kindly.)

Antonio knew the health costs of excessive alcohol and also the negative impact it was having on his marriage. But, as he reflected more deeply, he recognised further costs. For example, he slept poorly on nights when he drank heavily, which meant he woke up feeling sluggish and was less focused and more grumpy at work. On top of that, it was pulling him away from his core values of being loving and supportive as a partner, which in turn triggered guilt and anxiety.

5. What's the alternative?

It's easy to say 'I don't want to do XYZ any more'; it's much harder to say, 'Instead, I want to do ABC'. However, this is an essential step in breaking the habit. When those triggers are present — all those difficult situations, thoughts and feelings that you identified with question 2 — what are you going to do? If you're not going to do the behaviour you identified in question 1, what will you do instead? This is where you come back to your values: what values-based actions will you take?

Antonio identified that instead of drinking heavily he wanted to drink moderately: specifically, two bottles of beer a night instead of eight. So his new behaviour was to drink those two beers slowly, stretching them out over two hours, and then, once they were finished, to drink herbal tea or water for the rest of the night.

6. What skills can I use?

We can't change habits simply by thinking about it. The information we gathered in answering questions 1 to 5 is useful, but the real change happens with question 6 when we actively apply our ACT skills. Consider: what skills can you use to handle all those triggering thoughts, feelings, memories, sensations and urges? Dropping anchor, unhooking from your thoughts, making room for feelings, self-compassion, connecting with your values? Antonio used all of those skills to help him. As he drove home after work, he reminded himself of his values as a partner: loving, caring, supportive, patient, understanding. And when he got home, he waited 3 minutes before leaving his car. During that time, he dropped anchor, unhooked from his thoughts, and ran through his values again; then he opened up and made room for his feelings (including the urge to drink) and practised self-compassion. And throughout the evening, he used these skills over and over again, as often as he needed to. And as he flavoured his evenings with the values of self-care, being loving, and supportiveness — drinking sensibly, spending quality time with his wife — he actively savoured the difference this made in his life.

And did Antonio make these changes overnight? Did he do them perfectly? Did he stick to them ceaselessly? No, no and no. He most certainly did not. Why not? Because Antonio, like the rest of us, is a human being. And humans are imperfect; we are all flawed and fallible. We easily screw things up and let ourselves down. And when that happens, it's painful! Which is why we all need a lot more self-compassion.

The reality is, changing 'bad habits' takes time, and effort and energy, and it's rarely a smooth process. There'll be times we use our ACT skills, and they'll work well. There'll be other times we use them, and they won't work so well (because, hey, nothing is perfect). And there will be times we completely forget to use them, or can't be bothered using them, or don't even want to use them (because, hey, we're human). So we can expect ups and downs, break-throughs and set-backs, good patches and bad ones. That's the nature of changing our behaviour.

And it may take a long time before our new patterns become habitual — perhaps many months. So don't believe those books that tell you it only takes 21 days to form a new habit! There's no scientific basis for such claims. In my teens and twenties I was an extremely heavy drinker, whereas these days, I hardly drink at all. So 'drinking excessively' was a habit I successfully 'broke'. But 'unhealthy eating' — with a particular preference for chocolate, cake and ice-cream — is a habit I still struggle with intermittently. I go through periods where I successfully apply everything in this book, and I manage to eat pretty healthily. But I also go through phases where I stop applying ACT to this issue, and I fall back into unhealthy eating patterns and stack on the weight. In other words, some habits are easier to break than others.

Maintaining new habits

It's one thing to start some new type of life-enhancing behaviour; it's another thing to keep it going. So how can we sustain these new patterns until they really do become new habits? Well, there are hundreds, if not thousands of tools out there to help us with this challenge, but we can pretty much bundle them all into what

I like to call 'The Seven Rs': reminders, records, rewards, routines, relationships, reflecting and restructuring.

Let's take a look at each.

Reminders

We can create all sorts of simple tools to help remind us of our new behaviour. For example, we might create a pop-up or a screensaver on our computer or smartphone with an important word, phrase or symbol that reminds us to act mindfully or to utilise a particular value. We might use the old favourite of writing a message on a card and sticking it on the fridge, propping it against the bathroom mirror or taping it to the car dashboard. Or we might write something in a diary or calendar or in the 'notes' app of a smartphone. We might write just one word, like 'Breathe' or 'Pause' or 'Patience', or a phrase like 'Letting go' or 'Caring and compassionate'. Alternatively we might put a brightly coloured sticker on the strap of our wristwatch, the back of our smartphone or the keyboard of our computer, so that every time we use these devices the sticker reminds us to do the new behaviour.

Records

We can keep a record of our behaviour throughout the day, noting down when and where we do the new behaviour and what the benefits are; and also when and where we do the old behaviour and what the costs are. Any diary or notebook — on paper, or on a computer screen — can serve this purpose.

Rewards

When we do some form of new behaviour that involves acting on our values, hopefully that will be rewarding in its own right.

However, we can help to reinforce the new behaviour with additional rewards. One form of reward is kind, encouraging self-talk, e.g. saying to yourself: 'Well done. You did it!' Another form of reward is sharing your success and progress with a loved one who you know will respond positively. On the other hand, you might prefer more material rewards. For example, if you sustain this new behaviour for a whole week, you buy or do something that you really like, e.g. get a massage or buy a book.

Routines

If you get up every morning at the same time to exercise or do yoga, over time that regular routine will start to come naturally. You won't have to think so hard about doing it; it will require less 'willpower'; it will become a part of your regular routine. So experiment: see if you can find some way to build a regular routine or ritual around your new behaviour so it starts to become part of your way of life. For example, if you drive home from work, then every night, just before you get out of your car, you might do 2 minutes of dropping anchor, and reflect on what values you want to live by when you walk through the front door into your home.

Relationships

It's easier to study if you have a 'study buddy'; easier to exercise if you have an 'exercise buddy'. In AA programs, they team you up with a sponsor who is there to help you stay sober when the going gets tough. So can you find a kind, caring, encouraging person who can help support you with your new behaviour? Maybe you can check in with this person on a regular basis and tell them how well you are doing, as mentioned in 'Rewards'. Or maybe you can email your support person those records you've been keeping. Or maybe you can use the other person as a 'reminder'; ask them to remind you to do the new behaviour, if and when that would be useful. For example, you might say to your partner, 'When I raise my voice, can you please remind me to drop anchor?'

Reflecting

Regularly take time to reflect on how you are behaving and what effect it is having on your life. You can do this via writing it down — records — or in discussion with another person — relationships. Or you can do this as a mental exercise throughout the day, just before you go to bed, or just as you're waking up in the morning. You simply take a few moments to reflect on questions such as: 'How am I doing?', 'What am I doing that's working?', 'What am I doing that's not working?', 'What can I do more of, or less of, or differently?'

Make sure you also reflect on the times that you fall back into the old habit. Notice what triggers those relapses and setbacks, and notice what it costs you — i.e. how do you suffer? — when that happens. This doesn't mean beat yourself up! This means you non-judgmentally reflect on the genuine costs to your health and wellbeing of falling back into old habits — and use your awareness of the suffering this causes you to help motivate yourself to get back on track.

Restructuring

We can often restructure our environment to make our new behaviour easier, and therefore increase the chances we'll sustain it. For example, if the new behaviour is 'healthy eating' we can restructure the kitchen to make that easier: get rid of or hide away the junk food, and stock the fridge and pantry with the healthy stuff. If we want to go to the gym in the morning, we could pack up our sports gear in our gym bag and place it beside the bed or somewhere else obvious and convenient, so it's all ready to go as soon as we get up. (And of course, when we see our gym kit lying there, it acts as a reminder.)

So there you have it, 'The Seven Rs': reminders, records, rewards, routines, relationships, reflection, restructuring. Now be creative: mix and match these methods to your heart's content, to create your own set of tools for lasting change. Good luck with it!

Falling back into old habits

Whoever said 'practice makes perfect' was deluded. There's no such thing as perfection. Practice will help you establish better life skills — but it will not permanently eliminate all your self-defeating behaviours. You (and I, and everyone else on this planet) will screw up, make mistakes, and, at times, fall back into old habits. This will happen again and again and again. Indeed, because human beings screw up so often, I like to ask my clients two questions:

1. Next time you screw up, what would you ideally say or do to handle it more effectively?

2. If you have hurt yourself or others, what could you do to make amends and repair the damage?

Before answering these questions for yourself, get in touch with your values and reflect on the sort of person you want to be. If you could respond mindfully, acting on your core values, then what would you say and do when you notice you've screwed up? Are you willing to forgive yourself, let go, and move on? Are you willing to make room for your painful feelings, unhook from unhelpful thoughts, be kind to yourself and deal with the issue constructively, in a way that allows you to carry on with your life instead of getting bogged down in self-recrimination?

Note that this doesn't mean we're giving up. It just means we're being realistic. With practice, we can get much better at living by our values, engaging fully in life, practising forgiveness and self-compassion, unhooking from difficult thoughts, and making room for difficult feelings. So the more we practise, the better the outlook for the future. At the same time, we need to unhook from unrealistic expectations; to let go of trying to be perfect. The fact is, we will *not* always do what's most effective. We will *not* turn into saints or superheroes. We are human beings, which means we can never be perfect. No matter how much we apply the principles of ACT, and no matter how much they become 'second nature', there will be times when we forget and fall back into old ways.

That's why, when I counsel clients, I always discuss the issue of 'relapse'. I might say, 'Okay, so you just made a commitment that from now on, instead of yelling at your partner or your kids, you'll explain calmly and patiently why you're annoyed. Now I'm sure you're 100 per cent sincere about that; you certainly seem genuinely determined to work on this. My question is: how likely is it that you will never, ever yell at your loved ones — ever again?' In saying this, I'm not aiming to undermine their commitment; I am simply aiming to introduce some realism. I've found that most people appreciate this honesty. It helps them to loosen their grip on the 'Do It Perfectly' story.

The bottom line is: making changes is hard. We're all capable of doing it — *and* it's not easy. So set yourself up for success: small changes, baby steps, one brick at a time. And when you fall back into old habits (as you will) drop anchor, acknowledge the hurt, and hold yourself kindly.

PART 3
REVITALISE

19

THE STAGE SHOW OF LIFE

Tell me, what is it you plan to do with your
one wild and precious life?

—— *Mary Oliver*

I once heard a comedian say to a noisy heckler, 'Two hundred million sperm — and you had to be the one that got through!' When we think about it in these terms — that only one out of two hundred million sperm will successfully fertilise the egg — we realise we are pretty lucky to be alive. When you think about it even more broadly, and consider the chain of events that had to take place in order for you to be here — how your mother had to meet your father, and how their mothers and fathers had to meet each other, and so on, backwards to the dawn of life — it seems almost miraculous that you exist at all. In other words, we are privileged to be alive.

A 'privilege' means an advantage granted to a particular person or group. And an advantage is a condition or circumstance that puts us in a favourable position or provides us with a valuable opportunity. Each one of us is a member of a particular group that scientists refer to as *Homo sapiens*, and the fact that we are alive when so many members of our species are dead, puts us in a favourable position. It gives us a valuable opportunity to connect, care and contribute; to love and learn and grow. To treat life as a privilege means to seize that opportunity; to appreciate it, embrace it and savour it. In Chapter 7, I mentioned that when a reality slap involves death, or a close encounter with it, many of us experience a sense of doom or foreboding afterwards. We become acutely aware of the inevitability of death for each and every one of us. And often this triggers anxiety, vulnerability or insecurity. But if we explore those thoughts and feelings rather than pushing them away, we will discover they are telling us something important; they are reminding us that life is precious, and we are all vulnerable. We never know how long we have left to live, so we need to make the most of the time we have. We need to make the most of our one wild and precious life.

Of course, this is easy to say — but how do we actually do it? Well, if you've been applying the principles in this book you're already well on the way. Consider the idea that life is like a stage show, and on that stage are all your thoughts, emotions, memories, sensations and urges, along with everything you can see, hear, touch, taste and smell. This show changes continually, from moment to moment. And there's a part of you that can step back and watch it: zoom in and take in the details or zoom out and take in the big picture; dim the lights on side of the stage, or shine a spotlight on another.

We don't have a good word in everyday language for this part of you. When I'm in a poetic mood, I call it the 'observing self'; but most of the time I call it the 'part of you that notices'. You've been using this part of you for every mindfulness exercise throughout this book:

noticing your thoughts, noticing your feelings, noticing your body, noticing your actions, noticing the world around you. It's always there, always available, and you can utilise it in any moment to illuminate the aspects of the stage show you wish to explore. The show itself changes all the time. It's never the same in any two moments. At times, the stage seems full of pleasure and joy; but at other times it is crowded with hurt and misery.

When we receive a reality slap, the spotlight falls on our pain and the rest of the stage goes black, so it seems as if there is nothing to life but our suffering. But suppose we bring up the lights on the rest of the show. Suppose we illuminate *all* of the stage. Suppose we notice *both* our pain *and* all the life around it? (For no matter how great our pain, our life is larger.) What if, from that space of expansive awareness, we could notice the ways in which life is *not* lacking or damaged? And what if we could discover something very precious? What if we could find some hidden treasure that gives us a sense of fulfilment, even in the midst of our great pain?

Of course, our minds may say, 'While I have this problem/loss to deal with, nothing else matters' or 'Without X, Y or Z my life is empty/meaningless' or 'I don't care about anything else'. And if we get hooked by these thoughts, we will get lost in the smog: stumbling around, scarcely able to breathe. But if we want some relief from this smog, we can drop anchor, get present: unhook from those thoughts, cultivate awareness, and notice the *whole* of our life, not just the painful bits.

What might happen to your life if you were to notice all those things that most of us take for granted? And more than just notice them: *appreciate* them, *savour* them and *treasure* them? What if you were, in this moment, to treasure your breathing, or your eyesight, or your hearing, or the use of your arms and legs? What if you were to treasure your next encounter with friends, family or neighbours? Have you ever been for a walk and celebrated the beauty around you? Have you ever breathed in the air and rejoiced in its freshness? Have you ever relished the warmth of an open fire or a comfortable bed? Have you ever savoured a home-cooked meal, delighted in freshly baked bread or 'loved every minute' of a long hot shower? Have you ever found joy in a hug, or a kiss, or a book, or a movie, or a sunset, or a flower, or a child, or a pet?

At this point, your mind might be saying, 'Yeah, Russ, that's all very well, but what about those people who are stuck in truly horrific circumstances? Surely this isn't relevant to them?'

My answer is: first things first. When reality slaps us in the face, first we need to drop anchor and hold ourselves kindly. Next we need to take a stand: if we can't or won't leave, then we change what can be changed, accept what can't be changed, and live by our values. If we've done all that and the situation remains horrific then, yes, it'll probably be very hard to find anything to appreciate, savour or treasure. But it won't be impossible.

For example, in his autobiography, *Long Walk To Freedom*, Nelson Mandela describes how during his many years in prison on Robben Island he was able to savour his early morning marches to the quarry; to appreciate the fresh sea breeze and the beautiful wildlife. Or take the case of Primo Levi, an Italian Jew who was sent to Auschwitz concentration camp for the last year of World War II. In his moving book about that experience, *If This is a Man*, Levi describes how he endured backbreaking labour, day in day out, in the freezing Polish winter, wearing only the thinnest of clothes. But when the first days of spring appeared, he was able to truly savour the warmth of the sun. Finally, consider Viktor Frankl, another Jewish prisoner in Auschwitz. In his book, *Man's Search For Meaning*, he reveals how even in the midst of all that horror he was still able to treasure the sweet memories of his wife, from their life together before the atrocities started.

Notice I'm *not* suggesting we try to distract ourselves or pretend the reality slap never happened. I'm *not* saying we should look at all the other parts of the stage show and ignore those bits we don't like. I'm *not* proposing that we try to think positively and tell ourselves that this is all for the best. (You can try these approaches if you like, but for most of us they don't work very well — at least, not in the long term.) And I'm definitely *not* claiming this is going to get rid of your pain and make you feel happy!

What I *am* suggesting is simply this: let's bring up the lights on the *whole* stage show. Let's acknowledge all the difficulties, acknowledge all the painful thoughts and feelings — *and* also acknowledge the pleasures and wonders life gives us. Let's appreciate the privilege we have of simply being alive to witness this amazing stage show — and find something within it that we can treasure.

Of course, like many of the things in this book, this is much easier said than done. Why? Because the default setting of the human mind is to focus on what we *don't* have; on what's *not good enough*; on what needs to be fixed, solved or changed before we can appreciate life. This means that when someone starts talking about appreciating what we have, our minds may very well be cynical. So if your mind is now protesting, please treat it as if it's a loud voice in the far corner of a café: let it have its say, but don't get caught up in it or sucked into any kind of argument. And instead let's consider: how *can* we appreciate what we have?

The art of appreciation

It's actually quite simple to develop appreciation for the things we have. All we need to do is pay attention in a particular way: with openness and curiosity. Let's try it now. As you read this sentence, notice how your eyes are scanning the page; notice how they move from word to word without any conscious effort on your part; how they go at just the right speed for you to take in the information.

Now imagine how difficult life would be if you lost your eyesight. How much would you miss out on? Imagine if you could no longer read books, watch movies, discern the facial expressions of your loved ones, check out your reflection in a mirror, watch a sunset or drive a car.

Five things

When you reach the end of this paragraph, stop reading for a few seconds, look around and notice — and I mean *really notice* — five things you can see. Linger on each item for several seconds, noticing its shape, colour and texture, as if you are a curious child who has never seen anything like it. Notice any patterns or markings on the surface of these objects. Notice how the light reflects off them or the shadows they cast. Notice their contours, outlines and whether they are moving or still. Be open to the experience to discover something new, even if your mind insists it will be boring.

Then once you have finished, take a moment to consider just how much your eyes add to your life; consider what the gift of vision affords you. What would life be like if you were blind? How much would you miss out on?

This brief exercise brings together two important mindfulness skills: 'engaging' and 'savouring'. As we pay attention, with openness and curiosity, we *engage* in what we are doing; in other words, we become deeply involved in our experience. And as we truly appreciate our eyes and cherish the very miracle of vision itself, this gives rise to a sense of gratitude and fulfilment; in other words, we *savour* the experience.

Appreciating your hands

Now, as you continue reading, notice how your hands so effortlessly hold this book. When you get to the end of this paragraph, pick up the book, turn it upside down, flip it gently into the air and catch it. Spend a good minute or so playing with the book in different ways. Toss it from hand to hand, or flick through all the pages, or raise it up high and let it drop, catching it before it hits the ground. And, as you do these things, pay attention to the movements of your hands. Be curious about your hands: notice how they know exactly what to do; how the fingers and thumbs work so smoothly together. And be open to the experience; be open to learning from it, even if you really don't want to do it.

So, how amazing are your hands? How difficult would life be if you didn't have them? When you reach the end of the paragraph, use your hands to do something pleasant to yourself — gently stroke your scalp, massage your temples, rub your eyelids or massage a shoulder. Do this for a minute or so, slowly and gently, and again bring that childlike curiosity and openness to the process; notice how your hands move, and the sensations they generate, and the way your body responds.

Once you've done this, consider how much your hands contribute to your life and how much they enable you to do. Now try another exercise, which focuses on the breath.

Appreciating your breath

Now as you continue reading, slow your breathing. Take a few slow, deep breaths and let your shoulders drop. And as you appreciate the simple pleasure of breathing, reflect on the role your lungs play in your life. Consider how much you rely on them. Consider how much they contribute to your wellbeing. Millions of people all over the world have heart and lung diseases that make breathing very difficult, and if you've ever had asthma or pneumonia, you know just how difficult and scary that can be. Maybe you've visited someone in a hospital or a nursing home who was suffering from severe heart or lung disease; their lungs filling with fluid, the only way they could breathe was via inhaling oxygen through a mask. Imagine if that person were you. Imagine being in that situation and looking back over your life and remembering when your lungs once functioned well and how much easier your life was way back then. How much do we rely on our lungs and on our breath? And how often do we take these things for granted? Can you, just for a moment, notice your lungs in action and notice the breath flowing rhythmically — in and out — and savour the experience?

If we take the time throughout the day to slow down and appreciate what we have, we develop a greater sense of contentment. We can do this at any time and in any place: we simply take a few seconds to notice, with openness and curiosity, something we can see, hear, touch, taste or smell: perhaps the smile on the face of a loved one, or motes of dust dancing in a beam of sunlight, or the sensation of breath moving in and out of our lungs, or the sound of a child laughing, or the smell of brewing coffee, or the taste of butter on toast.

Now I'm not suggesting for a moment that this will solve all your problems. Nor am I asking you to pretend that everything in your life is hunky-dory and that you have no needs, wants and desires. The purpose of this practice is simply to increase our fulfilment. 'Finding the treasure' is a radically different psychological state to our default mindset of lack and discontentment and being fixated on trying to close or avoid the reality gap.

So, next time you drink some water, why not slow down a little and savour the first sip? Swill it once or twice around your mouth and notice how it instantly eases the dryness.

And next time you're out walking, why not take a few moments to notice the movement of your legs: their rhythm, strength and coordination, and appreciate the job they are doing of moving you around.

And next time you eat a delicious meal, why not savour the first mouthful and marvel at how your tongue is able to taste the food, and how your teeth are able to chew, and how your throat is able to swallow?

We all have a tendency to take life for granted, or to forget about all the wonder outside the reality slap. But it doesn't have to be that way. We don't have to wait until we're almost dying of thirst to appreciate the simple pleasure of drinking water. We don't have to wait until our legs stop working to appreciate how they carry us around. We don't have to wait until our eyes and ears fail to appreciate the gifts of vision and hearing. We can appreciate all these treasures, here and now.

20

THE FULL EXPERIENCE

Suppose you are in a lovely, cool, air-conditioned hotel room. You look out through the windows and gasp in admiration at a pristine white beach and the clear blue ocean, as far as the eye can see. The waves are sparkling in the sunlight and palm trees are swaying gently in the breeze. It's a truly spectacular view. But ... you cannot hear the pounding of the waves, you cannot feel the sunlight on your face, you cannot feel the breeze caressing your face, and you cannot breathe and smell the fresh sea air. This is what it's like to be 'half-present'. You take in some of your experience, but you miss out on a lot of it.

Now suppose you leave your room and step out onto the balcony. Instantly, you feel more alive. You can feel the kiss of sunlight on your skin, the wind gently tousling your hair and the fresh salty air filling your lungs. This is what it's like to be fully present, to engage in life as it is in this moment and soak up its richness, to drink it in and savour it. In the earlier sections of this book, we looked at mindfulness mainly as a means to reduce suffering: dropping anchor, making room for painful emotions, unhooking from difficult thoughts, and so on. We'll now explore a different aspect of mindfulness: using it to fully engage in life instead of taking it for granted.

Moments of engagement

Moments of engagement are natural. When we first meet someone we admire or find attractive, we are likely to be very engaged: we give them our full attention and we hang on their every word. And when we say someone has a 'strong presence' or that we find them 'engaging', what we mean is that they readily and naturally attract our attention. But what of those friends, family and colleagues whom we see all the time: how often do we take them for granted or only half-listen to them? We may even complain about how hard it is to stay present when they 'go on about things' and label them as 'boring'.

Similarly, when we taste the first mouthful of a delicious meal in a restaurant, or we smell some delightful new fragrance or set eyes upon a spectacular rainbow, for a moment or two we are likely to give it our full, conscious attention. But all too soon our attention wanes. After three or four mouthfuls of that meal, we start to take it for granted. Yes, we still taste it, but we are no longer savouring it, teasing out the tastes and exploring the textures. Instead, we are eating on autopilot, far more interested in the conversation with our dinner companions than in the sensations inside our mouth. And as for that beautiful fragrance: within minutes it fades into the background, until we hardly notice it any more.

Let's create some moments of engagement right now. In the exercise that follows, carry out each instruction for 5 to 10 seconds before moving on to the next.

Mindfulness of sounds

Firstly 'open your ears' and take a few moments to simply notice what you can hear.

Notice any sounds coming from you (e.g. your body moving in your chair, or your breathing).

Now 'stretch out your ears' to notice the sounds nearby.

Gradually expand your hearing range until you can hear the most distant sounds possible. Can you hear the sounds of the weather or the distant traffic?

Sit still in the midst of all this sound and notice the different layers: the vibrations, pulsations and rhythms.

Notice the sounds that stop and the new ones that start. See if you can notice a continuous sound of some sort, such as an electrical hum, or the whirring of a fan, and listen to it as if it's a piece of wondrous music. Notice the pitch, the volume and the timbre.

Stay with this noise and notice how it's not just 'one sound'. Notice there are layers within layers, rhythms within rhythms, and cycles within cycles.

Now notice the difference between the sounds you can hear and the words and pictures that your mind tries to attach to them.

How did you get on? Were you able to stay fully present with the sounds or did your mind pull you out of the exercise? Most of us find the latter. Did your mind perhaps distract you with thoughts like: 'This is boring', 'I can't do it', 'Why don't I skip this bit, I don't really need to do this' or 'What's for dinner?' Or did your mind perhaps conjure up images of the sounds you could hear — of people, cars, birds or the weather, for example? Or perhaps your mind had you analysing the sounds — 'I wonder what's making that noise?' — or had you identifying and labelling them — 'That's a truck'. Or maybe it just pulled you back to your reality gap: got you worrying about your problems or dwelling on how bad you feel, or wondering how this exercise can possibly help you. Whatever your mind did, it's quite okay; just notice that reaction and let it be.

Lisa and the frogs

'I can't stand it', said Lisa. 'If I have to listen to those bloody frogs for one more night, I swear I'll go crazy!' A week earlier, Lisa had moved into a lovely new house. Unfortunately, her next door neighbour had a large pond in her back garden, which was home to a family of exceedingly loud frogs. As Lisa described it, the frogs made a noise like two blocks of wood banging together, and they made it all night long. She found the noise intensely irritating and it kept her awake for hours. She'd tried three different types of earplugs, all to no avail, and she confessed — very guiltily — that she'd even started to think about poisoning the frogs.

I took her through the mindfulness of sounds exercise, and near the end of it I asked her to fix her attention on the somewhat irritating sound of a lawn mower, which was whirring loudly just across the road from my office. I asked her to be fully present with the sound: to let her mind chatter away in the background like a distant radio and to focus her attention on the sound itself; to notice, with great curiosity, all the different elements involved — the rhythms, vibrations, high notes, low notes, changes in pitch and volume — as if she were listening to the voice of a fabulous singer. Afterwards she reported that the noise quickly shifted from being annoying to rather interesting. She also expressed amazement that she had heard the sound of a lawnmower many hundreds of times, but she had never realised there was so much to it. So I asked her to practise this exercise in bed at night, to listen mindfully to the croaking frogs next door. A week later, she told me, with a huge grin on her face, that she had practised the exercise every night and she now enjoyed the sound of the frogs. She found it soothing and relaxing and it actually helped her drift off to sleep!

Now, I'd hate to set you up for unrealistic expectations: exercises like this don't always have such dramatic results, especially when we're new to them and our mindfulness skills are relatively undeveloped. Plus, let's not forget that staying present for long is hard to do, because our mind has so many clever ways of distracting us. So, if we want to get good at this, there is nothing for it but to practise. Therefore, I'd like to suggest two quick and simple exercises you could easily bring into your daily routine.

Mindfulness of people

Each day, pick one person and notice their face as if you've never seen it before: the colour of their eyes, teeth and hair, the pattern of the wrinkles in their skin and the manner in which they talk. Notice the way they move and walk, their facial expressions, body language and tone of voice. See if you can read their emotions and tune in to what they are feeling. When they talk to you, pay attention as if they are the most fascinating speaker you've ever heard and you've paid a million dollars for the privilege of listening. (Tip: Choose the person you will practise on the night before and then remind yourself of who it is first thing in the morning. This way, you're more likely to remember.) And very importantly: notice what happens as a result of this more mindful interaction.

Mindfulness of pleasure

Every day, pick a simple pleasurable activity — ideally one that you easily tend to take for granted or do on autopilot — and see if you can extract every last sensation of pleasure out of it. This might include hugging a loved one, stroking your cat, walking your dog, playing with your kids, drinking a cool glass of water or a warm cup of tea, eating your lunch or dinner, listening to your favourite music, having a hot bath or shower, walking in the park — you name it. (Note: Don't try this with activities that require you to get lost in your thoughts, such as reading, Sudoku, chess or crossword puzzles.) As you do this activity, use your five senses to be fully present: notice what you can see, hear, touch, taste and smell and savour every aspect of it.

Of course, there are an infinite number of practices that can help us develop the capacity to engage in and savour our experience. Why not invent some of your own? Basically, all you need to do is pick something — an object, activity or event — and give it your full, open, curious attention. Take in all the details through your five senses. And, at the same time, acknowledge how it contributes to your life.

And stay alert for that old 'Not Good Enough' story — it is always lurking in the background. And, if it hooks us, it's like a high-speed shuttle to hell. One moment, we're appreciating life here and now; the next we're deep in the bowels of the earth. Luckily, though, there is also a shuttle to heaven. As we unhook from unhelpful stories, make room for our difficult feelings and anchor ourselves firmly in the present, we ascend from the depths and come into the light. And when we go one step further and consciously appreciate what we have, we discover that our reality transforms. Our pain does not disappear, but it no longer dominates our attention; so, as well as acknowledging what we have lost, we can notice and appreciate what we have.

21

JOY AND SORROW

When one of my clients, Chloe, was diagnosed with breast cancer, she joined a so-called 'support group'. She had hoped to find a compassionate and self-aware community who could realistically acknowledge just how painful and scary and difficult cancer is, while also providing support and genuine encouragement. But what she found instead was, to use her terminology, 'a bunch of positive-thinking fanatics'. These women did not acknowledge Chloe's pain and fear. Instead they told her to think positively — to see her cancer as a 'gift'. They said she should consider herself lucky because this illness had given her a chance to 'wake up' and appreciate her life, a chance to learn and grow and love more fully.

Now, personally, I'm all for learning and growing and loving more fully, and this whole book is about waking up and appreciating life. But it's a big leap from that to seeing your cancer as a gift, or considering yourself lucky to have it. And replace the word 'cancer' with 'the death of your child', 'having your house burned down', 'sexual assault', 'living in a refugee camp' or 'losing your limbs'. How callous would it be to refer to these events as 'gifts' or to tell people they are 'lucky' when this happens? It is the very opposite of a caring and compassionate response.

All of us have plenty of opportunities to learn and grow and wake up and appreciate our lives; we don't need to have something terrible happen to us in order to do this. And if something terrible does happen, by all means let's learn and grow from it, but let's not pretend that it's wonderful or we're lucky to have it.

Having said that, from time to time you will meet or hear of someone who tells you that their illness, injury or near-death experience was the 'best thing that ever happened' to them because it transformed their life in such a positive way. I've met a couple of these folks, and I've read about quite a few others, and the genuine ones are truly inspiring; however, it seems to me that these people are extremely rare, and most of us will never see things the same way. So why not be honest with ourselves? When bad things happen, let's acknowledge how painful it is and be kind to ourselves. And then, and only then, let's consider how we might learn or grow from the experience.

So, if you *have* acknowledged your pain and responded to yourself with kindness, and done what you can to improve the situation, then it may *now* be time to consider several questions. Obviously you didn't ask for your reality slap to happen — life served it up without your consent — but given that it *has* happened, it may well be useful to ask yourself:

- How can I learn or grow from this experience?
- What personal qualities could I develop?
- What practical skills might I learn or improve?
- What strengths can I develop?
- What relationships can I deepen?

Every reality slap invites us to grow. We don't *want* that invitation, but if we turn it down, our life is sure to get worse. So how about we accept it and make the most of it? Let's use it to develop mindfulness and self-compassion, to get in touch with our values and act with purpose.

Part of the privilege of life is that we *do* have the opportunity to learn and grow, and we can make use of it any time, any place, right up until we take our final breath. So let's be curious: how can we deepen our life in response to distress? Can we perhaps develop more patience or courage? Or compassion, persistence or forgiveness?

Have you ever heard the old saying, 'When the student is ready, the teacher appears'? I used to cringe at this saying. I saw it as 'New Age' claptrap. I thought it meant that as soon as you were ready for the secret of enlightenment, some guru would magically appear out of thin air. But these days I interpret it very differently. I see it as meaning this: if we are willing to learn, we can do so from literally anything life dishes up. No matter how painful or scary it may be, we can always learn something useful from it.

Now suppose I say to you 'I've got this gadget' and I pull out a little silver box with a bright red button on top. And I say to you 'This device is amazing. All you need to do is press this red button and all your fear, anger, guilt, loneliness and sadness will completely disappear. So will all those painful memories. In fact, you'll never experience pain ever again. There's only one side effect. When you press that button, you won't care about anyone or anything. You won't care about your friends, partner or family; you won't care if they're happy or sad, if they live or die. You won't care about your career, your house, your neighbourhood, your country, the planet; you won't care about anything that happens, ever. You'll have no goals, no desires, no wishes. Your life will lack any sense of meaning or purpose, because you care about absolutely nothing. But, hey, there will be no more pain.'

Would you press that button?

This is what life gives us. If we're going to care about anyone or anything at all, then sooner or later we will encounter a gap between what we want and what we've got. And the bigger that gap, the greater our pain. *Those things that truly matter also hurt.*

So can we make room for those painful feelings and see them as a valuable part of us? Can we appreciate that they tell us something important: that we are alive, we have a heart, and we truly care?

Can we see our pain as a bridge to the hearts of others? That it spans our differences and unites us in the commonality of human suffering. Only when we know what it's like to hurt can we relate well to others who are suffering; only then will we understand the true meaning of empathy. So, can we appreciate how pain helps us to build rich relationships, to *connect* with the pain of others, to actively *care* about them and to willingly *contribute* kindness when they are hurting?

Our emotions are as much a part of us as our arms and our legs. So, do we really have to avoid, escape or fight them? When our arms and legs get cut, broken or infected, naturally they give rise to pain. But we don't get into a fight with our limbs because of it, or wish we could go through life without them. We appreciate what they contribute to our life.

So, let's now consider that part of us which cares. What if we could truly treasure this part and truly be grateful for all it affords us in life? Yes, if we didn't care we'd have no pain, but we'd also have no joy or love or laughter. We'd go through life like zombies; everything would be pointless or meaningless. There would be no disappointment or frustration, but there would also be no contentment or satisfaction. Our capacity to care enables us to live a life of purpose: to build rich relationships, to motivate ourselves, to find life's treasures and enjoy them. So, can we be grateful for it, even though it brings us so much pain?

Let's also consider our ability to *feel* emotions. Can we appreciate the brain's amazing ability to take billions of electrochemical signals coming in from all over the body and decode them and interpret them in an instant, to enable us to feel whatever we feel?

Just imagine if this system didn't work. Imagine if we felt nothing ever again. How much would we miss out on? How empty would life be?

From a mental viewpoint of self-compassion, having dropped anchor and taken a purposeful stand, can we look at these painful feelings inside our body and treat them with kindness and respect? Can we give them space, and give them peace, and give them our caring attention? Can we reflect on how they remind us of what we care about? Can we let go of judging these feelings as 'bad' and instead cultivate wonder that they exist at all?

I've saved this chapter for the end because it's the hardest thing I am suggesting in this book. To tolerate pain is difficult; to accept it is much harder. But to appreciate it is the hardest challenge of all.

And yet, it is possible. The more we reflect on the privilege of human emotion — that we get to care and to feel in so many different ways — the more we can appreciate *all* our emotions. Yes, this privilege does not come without a price. With passion comes pain. With caring comes loss. With wonder comes fear and dread.

The famous Lebanese author, Kahlil Gibran, expressed these ideas wonderfully in his amazing book of poetry, *The Prophet*. Here's an extract:

The Reality Slap

Joy and Sorrow

Your joy is your sorrow unmasked.

And the selfsame well from which your laughter rises was oftentimes
filled with your tears.

And how else can it be?

The deeper that sorrow carves into your being, the more joy you
can contain.

Is not the cup that holds your wine the very cup that was burned in
the potter's oven?

And is not the lute that soothes your spirit, the very wood that was
hollowed with knives?

When you are joyous, look deep into your heart and you shall find it is
only that which has given you sorrow that is giving you joy.

When you are sorrowful look again in your heart, and you shall see
that in truth you are weeping for that which has been your delight.

Some of you say, 'Joy is greater than sorrow,' and others say,
'Nay, sorrow is the greater.'

But I say unto you, they are inseparable.

Together they come, and when one sits alone with you at your board,
remember that the other is asleep upon your bed.

Life is a great privilege, and the challenge for all of us is to make the most of it. Can we let our values guide us, can we treat ourselves kindly, make room for both our sorrow and our joy, and engage fully in the great and everchanging stage show of life? For sure, we can. And, at the same time, we need to be realistic: the inconvenient truth is that we will often forget to do this. But, the beautiful thing is, whenever we *do* remember, we have a choice. We can hold ourselves kindly, drop anchor, and take a stand. And right there, in that moment, we can find treasure; it's always there, even when life hurts.

APPENDIX A:
NEUTRALISATION

Neutralising your thoughts means putting them into a new context where you can readily recognise that they are constructs of words and pictures; this neutralises their power.

Neutralisation techniques typically involve either highlighting the visual properties of thoughts (i.e. 'seeing' them) or the auditory properties of thoughts (i.e. 'hearing' them), or both. I encourage you to experiment with the techniques that follow and be curious as to what will happen. You can't accurately predict in advance which techniques will work best for you. Some may work really well, others not at all. (And sometimes a technique backfires and gets you even more hooked than before; this is uncommon, but it does occasionally happen.)

Keep in mind that the purpose of unhooking is *not* to get rid of unwanted thoughts, nor to reduce unpleasant feelings. The aim *is* to enable you to engage fully in life instead of getting lost in or pushed around by your thoughts. When we defuse from unhelpful thoughts, we often find that they quickly 'disappear', or our unpleasant feelings rapidly reduce — but such outcomes are 'lucky bonuses', not the main aim. So by all means enjoy these things when they happen, but don't expect them — or you will soon be disappointed.

I invite you to try out the following techniques and be curious about what happens. If you find one or two that really help you to unhook, play around with them over the next few weeks and see what difference it makes. However, if any of these techniques make you feel trivialised or mocked, then do *not* use them.

Visual neutralisation techniques

First, on a piece of paper, jot down several of the thoughts that most frequently hook you and distress you. For each technique below, pick one of these thoughts to work with, go step-by-step through the exercise, and be curious about and open to whatever happens.

Thoughts on paper

Write two or three distressing thoughts on a large piece of paper. (If you don't have access to paper and pens right now, you can try doing this exercise in your imagination.)

Now hold the piece of paper in front of your face and get absorbed in those distressing thoughts for a few seconds.

Next, place the paper down on your lap, look around you, and notice what you can see, hear, touch, taste and smell.

Notice the thoughts are still with you. Notice they haven't changed at all, and you know exactly what they are, but do they somehow have less impact when you rest them on your lap instead of holding them in front of your face?

Now pick up the paper and, underneath those thoughts, draw a stick figure (or, if you have an artistic streak, some sort of cartoon character). Draw a 'thought bubble' around those words, as if they are coming out of the head of your stick figure (just like those thought bubbles you see in comic strips). Now look at your 'cartoon': does this make any difference to the way you relate to those thoughts?

Try this a few times with different thoughts and stick figures (or cartoons). Put different faces on your stick figures — a smiley face, a sad face, or a face with big teeth or spiky hair. Draw a cat, or a dog, or a flower, with those very same thought bubbles coming out of it. What difference does this make to the impact of those thoughts? Does it help you to see them as words?

Computer screen

You can do this exercise in your imagination or on a computer. (For most people it's more powerful to do it on a computer.) First write (or imagine) your thought in standard black lower-case text on the computer screen, then play around with the font and the colour. Change it into several different colours, fonts and sizes, and notice what effect each change makes. (Note: bold red capitals are likely to cause fusion for most people, whereas a lower-case pale pink font is more likely to create defusion.)

Then change the text back to black and lower-case, and this time play around with the formatting. Space the words out, placing large gaps between them.

Run the words together with no gaps between them so they make one long word.

Run them vertically down the screen.

Then put them back together as one sentence.

How do you relate to those thoughts now? Is it easier to see that they are words? (Remember, we are not interested in whether the thoughts are true or false; we just want to see them for what they are.)

Karaoke ball

Imagine your thought as words on a karaoke screen. Imagine a 'bouncing ball' jumping from word to word across the screen. Repeat this several times.

If you like, you can even imagine yourself up on stage singing along to the words on the screen.

Changing scenarios

Imagine your thought in a variety of different settings. Take about 5 to 10 seconds to imagine each scenario, then move on to the next one. See your thought written:

- in playful colourful letters on the cover of a children's book
- as stylish graphics on a restaurant menu
- as icing on top of a birthday cake
- in chalk on a blackboard
- as a slogan on the T-shirt of a jogger.

Leaves on a stream or clouds in the sky

Imagine leaves gently floating down a stream, or clouds gently floating through the sky. Take your thoughts, place them on those leaves or clouds, and watch them gently float on by.

Auditory neutralisation techniques

These auditory neutralisation techniques give you more opportunities to place your thoughts in a different context. Experiment with them and notice what happens.

Silly voices

Say your thought to yourself in a silly voice — either silently or out loud. (It is generally more defusing to do it out loud, but obviously you need to pick the time and place; it doesn't go down well in a business meeting!) For example, you might choose the voice of a cartoon character, movie star, sports commentator or someone with an outrageous foreign accent. Try several different voices and notice what happens.

Slow and fast

Say your thought to yourself — either silently or out loud — first in ultra slow motion, then at superfast speed (so you sound like a chipmunk).

Singing

Sing your thoughts to yourself — either silently or out loud — to the tune of *Happy Birthday*. Then try it with a couple of different tunes.

Create your own neutralisation techniques

Now invent your own neutralisation techniques. All you need to do is put your thought in a new context where you can 'see' it or 'hear' it, or both. For example, you might visualise your thought painted on a canvas, printed on a postcard, emblazoned on the chest of a comic book superhero, carved on the shield of a medieval knight, trailed on a banner behind an aeroplane, tattooed on the back of a biker, or written on the side of a zebra among all its stripes. Or you could paint it, draw it or sculpt it. Or you could imagine it dancing, or jumping, or playing football. Or you could visualise it moving down a TV screen, like the credits of a movie. Alternatively, you might prefer to imagine hearing your thought being recited by a Shakespearean actor, broadcast from a radio, emanating from a robot or sung by a rock star. You are limited only by your own creativity, so be sure to play around and have some fun.

APPENDIX B:

MINDFULNESS OF THE BREATH

This exercise is very useful for developing your mindfulness skills. (In *The Reality Slap: Extra Bits* there's a free audio recording of the exercise.) Before commencing, decide how long you are going to spend on this practice — 10 to 20 minutes is ideal, but you can do it for as little or as long as you wish. (It's generally a good idea to use a timer of some sort.) Also, keep in mind that a very small number of people have unpleasant reactions when focusing on the breath, such as dizziness, pins and needles, or anxiety; if this happens for you, stop the exercise.

Find a quiet place where you are free from any distractions such as pets, children and phone calls, and get yourself into a comfortable position, ideally sitting up in a chair or on a cushion. (Lying down is okay, but it's very easy to fall asleep!) If you are sitting, straighten your back and let your shoulders drop. Then, close your eyes or fix them on a spot. (It's easier to stay awake if your eyes are open.)

For the first few breaths, focus on gently emptying your lungs; ever so slowly, exhale until your lungs are completely empty. Then pause for a second, and then allow them to fill by themselves, from the bottom up.

After five or six of these breaths, allow your breathing to find its own natural pace and rhythm; there is no need to control it.

Your challenge for the rest of the exercise is to keep your attention on the breath; to observe it as if you are a curious child who has never encountered breathing before. As your breath flows in and out, notice the different sensations you feel in your body.

Notice what happens in your nostrils.

Notice what happens in your shoulders.

Notice what happens in your chest.

Notice what happens in your abdomen.

With openness and curiosity, track the movement of your breath as it flows through your body; follow the trail of sensations in your nose, shoulders, chest and abdomen.

As you do this, let your mind chatter away like a radio in the background: don't try to silence it, you'll only make it louder. Simply let your mind chatter away and keep your attention on the breath.

From time to time, your mind will hook you with thoughts and feelings, and pull you out of the exercise. This is normal and natural — and it will keep happening. (Indeed, you're doing well if you last even 10 seconds before it happens!)

Once you realise you've been hooked, gently acknowledge it. Silently say to yourself, 'Hooked', or gently nod your head and refocus on your breath.

This 'hooking' will happen again and again and again, and each time you unhook yourself and return your attention to the breath you are building your ability to focus. So if your mind hooks you one thousand times, then one thousand times you acknowledge it and refocus on your breathing.

As the exercise continues, the feelings and sensations in your body will change: you may notice pleasant ones, such as relaxation, calmness and peace, or uncomfortable ones, such as backache, frustration or anxiety. The aim is to allow your feelings to be as they are, regardless of whether they are painful or pleasant.

Remember, this is *not* a relaxation technique. You are not trying to relax. It's quite all right if you feel stressed, anxious, bored or impatient. Your aim is to allow your feelings to be as they are in this moment — without a struggle.

So if a difficult feeling is present, silently name it: say to yourself, 'Here's boredom' or 'Here's frustration' or 'Here's anxiety'. Let it be and keep your attention on the breath.

Continue in this way — observing the breath, acknowledging uncomfortable feelings, unhooking yourself from thoughts — until you reach the end of your allotted time.

Then have a good stretch, engage with the world around you, and congratulate yourself on taking the time to practise this valuable life skill.

APPENDIX C:
GOAL SETTING

Effective goal setting is quite a skill and it does require a bit of practice to get the hang of it.

The method that follows is adapted with permission from the book *The Weight Escape* by Ann Bailey, Joe Ciarrochi and Russ Harris. You can download this worksheet from the free eBook: *The Reality Slap: Extra Bits*.

The five-step plan for goal setting and committed action

Step 1: Identify your guiding values
Identify the value or values that will underpin your course of action.

_____

_____

_____

_____

_____

_____

_____

Step 2: Set a SMART goal

It's not effective to set any old goal that springs to mind. Ideally, you want to set a SMART goal. Here's what the acronym means:

S = specific. Do not set a vague, fuzzy or poorly-defined goal like, 'I'll be more loving'. Instead, be specific: 'I'll give my partner a good, long hug when I get home from work'. In other words, specify what actions you will take.

M = motivated by values. Make sure this goal is aligned with your chosen values.

A = adaptive. Is it wise to pursue this goal? Is it likely to make your life better?

R = realistic. Make sure the goal is realistic for the resources you have available. Resources could include: time, money, physical health, social support, knowledge and skills. If these resources are necessary but unavailable, you will need to change your goal to a more realistic one. The new goal might actually be to find the missing resources: to save the money, or develop the skills, or build the social network, or improve health, etc.

T = timeframed. Put a specific timeframe on the goal. Specify the day, date and time — as accurately as possible — that you will take the proposed actions.

Write your SMART goal here:

_____

_____

_____

_____

_____

_____

_____

Step 3: Identify benefits

Clarify for yourself, what would be the most positive outcome(s) of achieving your goal? (However, *don't* start fantasising about how wonderful life will be after you achieve your goal; research shows that fantasising about the future actually reduces your chances of following through!) Write the benefits below:

_____

_____

_____

_____

_____

_____

_____

Step 4: Identify obstacles

Imagine the potential difficulties and obstacles that might stand in the way of you achieving your goals, and how you will deal with them if they arise. Consider:

- what are the possible *internal* difficulties (difficult thoughts and feelings, such as low motivation, self-doubt, distress, anger, hopelessness, insecurity, anxiety, etc.)?

- what are the possible *external* difficulties (things aside from thoughts and feelings that might stop you, e.g. lack of money, lack of time, lack of skills, personal conflicts with other people involved)?

If internal difficulties arise in the form of thoughts and feelings, such as:

_____

_____

then I will use the following mindfulness skills to unhook, make room and get present:

_____

_____

If external difficulties arise, such as:

a)_____

b)_____

c)_____

then I will take the following steps to deal with them:

a)_____

b)_____

c)_____

Step 5: Make a commitment

Research shows that if you make a public commitment to your goal (i.e. if you state your goal to at least one other person) you are far more likely to follow through on it. If you're not willing to do this, then at the very least make a commitment to yourself. But if you really *do* want the best results, then make your commitment to somebody else you trust.

I commit to (*write your values-guided SMART goal here*):

_____

_____

_____

_____

_____

_____

_____

_____

Now say your commitment out loud — ideally to someone else, but if not, to yourself.

Other helpful tips for goal setting

Make a step-by-step plan: break your goal down into concrete, measurable and time-based sub-goals.

Tell other people about your goal and your ongoing progress: making a public declaration increases commitment.

Reward yourself for making progress in your goal: small rewards help push you on to major success. (A reward might be as simple as saying to yourself, 'Well done! You made a start!')

Record your progress: keep a journal, graph or drawing that plots your progress.

RESOURCES

Free eBook: The Reality Slap: Extra Bits

This eBook (a pdf) contains links to download many free audio recordings, plus a few additional resources to support the main book. You can download it from the 'Free resources' page on www.thehappinesstrap.com.

Other books by Russ Harris

The Happiness Trap: Stop struggling, start living

Many popular notions of happiness are misleading, inaccurate and will actually make you miserable if you believe them. *The Happiness Trap* is a self-help book written for everyone and anyone on how to make life richer, fuller and more meaningful, while avoiding common 'happiness traps'. Based on ACT (Acceptance and Commitment Therapy), it is applicable to everything from work stress and addictions, to anxiety and depression, to the pressures of parenting and the challenges of terminal illness. Widely used by ACT practitioners and their clients all around the world, *The Happiness Trap* has sold over one million copies, and been translated into over thirty languages. Go to the

'Free resources' page on www.thehappinesstrap.com for many useful materials to use with the book.

ACT with Love

This inspiring and empowering self-help book teaches you how to apply the principles of ACT to common relationship issues, and shows how to move from conflict, struggle and disconnection to forgiveness, acceptance, intimacy and genuine loving.

The Confidence Gap

Is there a gap between where you are right now and where you want to be? Is a lack of confidence holding you back? We've all been stuck in the 'confidence gap': we want to find a better job, pursue a romantic relationship, enrol in a course, expand our business, or pursue our greatest dreams, but fear, doubt or insecurity gets in the way and we don't take action. Russ Harris has helped thousands of people overcome fear and develop genuine confidence, using the principles of ACT — and this book reveals how it is done. Compassionate, practical and inspiring, *The Confidence Gap* will help you identify your passions, succeed at your challenges and create a life that is truly fulfilling.

ACT Made Simple: An easy-to-read primer on Acceptance and Commitment Therapy (2nd ed.)

This practical and entertaining textbook for psychologists, counsellors, therapists and coaches is equally useful for experienced ACT practitioners and total newcomers to the approach. *ACT Made Simple* offers clear explanations of the core ACT processes and real-world tips and solutions for rapidly and effectively implementing them in your coaching or therapy practice. Reading this book is all the training you need to begin using ACT techniques with your clients for impressive results.

Audio MP3s by Russ Harris

Mindfulness Skills: volumes 1 and 2

Available as downloadable MP3 files, these two volumes cover a wide range of mindfulness exercises for personal use. You can get them via the online store on www.actmindfully.com.au.

'In person' and online ACT training for health professionals

ACT training for therapists, coaches, counsellors, doctors, nurses, social workers, psychologists, psychiatrists, youth workers and occupational therapists.

Russ Harris provides a wide range of professional training workshops in person in Australia, but you can access his training and advice through online courses, too. For online courses, see www.ImLearningACT.com.

The Happiness Trap: online self-help program

Have you tried hard to be happier and found it just wasn't that easy? If so, that's hardly surprising. Commonplace notions of happiness are misleading, inaccurate and can actually make you miserable. So come along and learn about *happiness without all the hype*. Learn how to 'escape the happiness trap' and find genuine wellbeing and fulfilment. This entertaining and empowering online program, written and presented by Russ Harris, is based on his international bestseller *The Happiness Trap*. To find out more go to www.thehappinesstrap.com.

Facebook groups — public and professional

If you're a health professional (of any sort) check out the 'ACT Made Simple' Facebook group. Tens of thousands of health practitioners from around the world ask questions, provide answers and share resources about anything and everything to do with the professional use of ACT in counselling, coaching and therapy.

If you're using ACT for self-help or personal growth, join the 'Happiness Trap Online' Facebook group. It's a private group where we can all share our struggles and explore how to use ACT with them.

ACKNOWLEDGMENTS

First and foremost, I am deeply indebted and incredibly grateful to my partner, Natasha, for all her love and support while I was writing this book (as well as all her love and support when I was not writing the book!).

Next, a planet-sized amount of thanks to Steven Hayes, the originator of ACT, for not only introducing this amazing model to the world, but also for all his help and encouragement with my books and my career. And that gratitude also extends to the larger ACT community worldwide, which is always very supportive and giving and caring.

Thirdly, a huge amount of gratitude goes to my agent, Sammie Justesen, for all her continuing good work.

Fourthly, my thanks to Joe Ciarrochi and Ann Bailey for allowing me to use the goal-setting materials we created for *The Weight Escape*.

And, last but not least, several truckloads of thanks to the entire team at Exisle Publishing — especially Gareth Thomas, Anouska Jones and Karen Gee — for all the hard work, care and attention they have invested.

INDEX

A

A kind hand exercise 118–19

acceptance, stage of grief 4, 5

ACE formula

    explained 46–7

    in practice 47–50

acknowledgment, thoughts and
    feelings 47

ACT (Acceptance and
    Commitment Therapy)

    explained 8–10

    titles 247–9

    titles for health
    professionals 249

    WHO program 10

alcohol

    moderating level 196–7

    'self-care' 19

    unhooking from 181–2

Ali, PTSD 53–4

anchor dropping

    aims 50

effect of 99

exercises 46–57

anger

    motivation of 93

    stage of grief 4, 5

Antonio

    acknowledging pain
    29–30

    changing behaviour
    patterns 196–7

    dealing with SIDS 24–6

    dropping anchor 55

    'giving support' to self 134

    grieving practice 133

    rebuilding his life 165–6

    Speak kindly exercise
    122–3

    words for pain 31–2

    words of kindness 32–3

anxiety, motivation of 94

any time, any place exercise
    55–7

appreciation, art of naming
210–13
audio MP3s 249
auditory neutralisation
techniques 235–6
avoidance, of other people
14–17
awareness, expanding 112–14

B
'bad habits'
changing patterns 192–7
common payoffs 194
falling back into 201–2
patterns of 191–2
bargaining 4, 5
bear, fighting off 6–7
behaviour, new habits 192–7
blaming 64
blue-ringed octopus
faced with 101–3
painful emotion analogy
102
body
connection with 48–9,
55–6, 163
cut off from 97
distractions 95–7
book experiment 42–4
breathing
appreciating 212–13

mindfulness 117–18,
237–9
and spirituality 85–6
into your feelings 110–11
breathing exercises 85–90,
107, 110–11

C
cancer
author's father's story
186–7
joy and sorrow 223–4
Cathy, grieving practice 133
challenge formula
options 171–8
realities of choices 175–6
children, expressing emotions
37–8
classroom behaviour, without
teacher 97–8
comfort eating 19
'common humanity' 126
communication, with others
92–3
computer screen exercise
233–4
connection
limits on 16
and reflect exercise 154–6
with your body 48–9,
55–6, 163

control
    focus on what you can
    13–14
    by our emotions 37–8
    strategies 114
coping methods 17–18
creative pursuits 20
curiosity, role in emotional
    healing 106

D
Dave, rebuilding his life 166–7
death
    talking with loved one 129
    thoughts of 80–1
deformities, looking past 105
denial 4, 5
depression, stage of grief 4, 5
disconnection, side effects of
    97
distractions, strategies 38–9
donkey, carrot vs stick 115–16
doom and death anxiety 65
dropping anchor see anchor
    dropping

E
Emily, self-support 134
emotional disconnection 97
emotional pain see pain
emotional storms

anchors don't control
    50–2
fight, flight or freeze
    response 52–3
handling 46–57
emotions
    ACE formula 46–50
    allowing 111–12
    avoidance of 106
    awareness of 97–8
    breathing into 110–11
    children expressing 37–8
    clarifying 103–7
    control strategies 114
    controlled by 37–8
    cut off from 98
    expanding awareness
    112–14
    experience full range 39
    illumination of 94–5
    making room for 107–14
    naming exercise 110
    notice your feeling 108–110
    painful 104–5
    three main purposes 92–5
engagement, moments of 216
exercises
    anchor-dropping 46–57
    approach to 107–8
    book experiment 42–4

breathing 85–90, 107, 110–11
computer screen 233–4
connect and reflect 154–6
connect with body 48–9
'giving support' 134–9
karaoke ball 234
kindness 118–23
'letting go' 86–90
mindful breathing 237–40
mindfulness 117–28, 217–20, 237–9
mindfulness of people 219
mindfulness of pleasure 220
mindfulness of sounds 217–19
naming 77–8
naming the story 79–81
noticing five things 210–11
practising ACE formula 47–50
self-judgements 149–56
self-kindness 35–7
silly voices 235
Speak kindly exercise 122–3
values 145–7
values vs goals 147–54
voice techniques 235

writing thoughts 232–3
experiments
  unhooking from thoughts 72–3
  using a book 42–4

F
Facebook groups 250
fear 93, 94
feelings see emotions
fibromyalgia
  effect of 15
  limitations with 19–20
  limited activities 151–2
  rebuilding life 167–8
  self-critical thoughts 70–1
  words expressing pain 32
fight, flight or freeze response 5–8, 45, 53, 56, 92, 99
five things, noticing 210–11
flashbacks 53–4
focus, on what's in your control 13–14, 175–6
foreboding 65
forgiveness
  notion of 180
  practising 181–3
Frankl, Viktor 209

G
Gibran, Kahlil 227–8

goal setting, five-step plan
241–5
goals
SMART 242–3
vs values 147–54
grief
creating practice of 132
five stages 4–5
groundwork 129–30
guilt 93, 94, 95

H
hands, appreciating 211
Harris, Dr Russ (author)
father's illness 186–7
own reality slaps 9
WHO ACT program 10
hobbies 20
Hold yourself kindly exercise
121
hopelessness 63

I
inner voices, battling them
66–7
insecurity 64
intimacy, emotional/
psychological 185–8

K
karaoke ball exercise 234

kindness
acts of 113
needed from self 23–4
words to self 32–6
kindness exercises 118–23
Kübler-Ross, Dr Elisabeth 4–5

L
leprosy 91–2
'letting go' exercise 86–90
Levi, Primo 208–9
life
adding meaning to 143–5
privilege of 205–9, 225–9
rebuilding 164–8
six months from now
156–7
lifelessness, sense of 96
Lisa, and the frogs 218–19
loss
acknowledging 130–4
talking with loved one
132–4
love 93, 94, 95

M
Mandela, Nelson 174, 208
Mandela University 174
meaning, sense of 143–4
meaninglessness 63

memories
  choosing 132
  mixed emotions 129
  remembering and allowing 131
Michael, unhooks from alcohol 181–2
mind
  thanking yours 82
  what it does 61–4
mindfulness
  appreciating simple pleasures 210
  breathing 117–18, 237–9
  explained 117–18
  noticing five things 210–11
  of people 219
  of pleasure 220
  of sounds 217–19
missing out 95–7
motivation
  underlying activities 144–5
  various emotions 93–4
movies, with sound off 98

N
naming exercise 77–8
naming the pattern 78–9
naming the story 79–81
Natalie
  'bad mother' story 150–1

expressing pain 32
rebuilding her life 167
words for pain 32
words of kindness 33
nature walks 17–18
Neff, Kristin
  expressing self-compassion 32
  self-compassion core elements 126
  words of kindness 32
neutralisation techniques
  auditory 235
  creating own 236
  explained 82–3
  visual 232–5
'Not Good Enough' stories 29

O
'observing self' 206–9
obstacles, identifying 243–4
Open up exercise 119–20
oxygen mask, putting on 28

P
pain
  ability to eliminate 225–6
  acknowledging 29–34
  relief strategies 38–40
  serves a purpose 92

words expressing 29–30
painful emotion analogy 102
parents, feelings about children 41
past, dwelling on 62
patterns
  breaking 158
  naming 78–9
  triggers 193
payoffs, behaviour patterns 193–4
physical activities 19
pointlessness 63
progress, reflecting on 199
psychological smog
  acknowledging 59–73
  caught up in 67–8
PTSD (post-traumatic stress disorder) 54

R
Rada
  effect of fibromyalgia 15
  expressing pain 32
  fibromyalgia limitations 15
  rebuilding her life 167–8, 175
  regaining activities 151–3
  self-critical thoughts 70–1
  words expressing pain 32

words of kindness 32–3
reaching out 16
realism, what you can do 175–6
reality slap
  reactions to 8–9
  response options 41–4
reason-giving 63
records 198
reflection, exercise 155–6
refugee camps, WHO program 175
relationships
  challenge options 172–5
  examining your own 157–9
  support person 199–200
reminders 198
resentment 64, 179–83
restructuring 200–1
revenge 60
rewards 198–9
road traffic noise 71–2
routines 199
rules vs values 177–8
ruminating 62

S
sadness 93, 94, 95
scenarios, changing patterns 234

screwing up, response to
115–16
self-blame, resentment as
180–1
self-care
a balancing act 19–21
kindness 23–4
self-compassion
attitude towards 27–8
core elements 126–8
defined 27–8
kindness exercises 118–23
self-criticism
harsh thoughts 78
mind's involvement 62–3
self-defeating behaviour,
changing patterns
191–202
self-doubt 64
self-pity 28
self-talk
kindness 23–36
responding to 124–5
sensations, clarifying 103–7
Shanti
anchor-dropping exercise
52
grieving ritual 133–4
pain of betrayal 37
rebuilding her life 166

SIDS
dealing with 24–6
silly voices exercise 235
sleep, disrupted 19
SMART goals 242–3
Speak kindly exercise 122–3
spirituality, and breathing
85–6
sports 20
Stevenson, Robert Louis 57
stories
in the mind 61–5
naming exercise 79–81
suicidality 64
survivor guilt 24
symbolic acts 131

T
terminal illness 81–2
The Reality Slap: Extra Bits
(free eBook) 10, 50, 237,
241
'The Seven Rs' (habit-changing
tools) 197–201
thoughts
art of naming 76
controlling difficult ones
42–4
of death 80–1
explained 68–72
helpful 81

naming the pattern
78–9
neutralising 82–3
smoky haze 67–8
unhooking from 69–72
writing down 232–3
triggers, behaviour patterns
193

V
values
examining your own
156–9
exercise 145–7
vs goals 147–54
personal 144–7
vs rules 177–8
visual neutralisation
techniques 232–6
vitality 96
voices, 'inner critic' 59–61
vulnerability 65

W
websites, free resources 10,
247, 248
WHO program, refugee camps
175
willingness 176–8
withdrawal, from other people
14–17
words
distraction 96
expressing pain 29–30
of kindness 32–6
spiritual tradition 85
vitality 96
worrying 62
worst, predicting 62

Y
'younger you' 135–8

Z
Zen masters 66